Methods in Molecular Biology

Series Editor
John M. Walker
School of Life and Medical Sciences
University of Hertfordshire
Hatfield, Hertfordshire, UK

For further volumes:
http://www.springer.com/series/7651

For over 35 years, biological scientists have come to rely on the research protocols and methodologies in the critically acclaimed *Methods in Molecular Biology* series. The series was the first to introduce the step-by-step protocols approach that has become the standard in all biomedical protocol publishing. Each protocol is provided in readily-reproducible step-by-step fashion, opening with an introductory overview, a list of the materials and reagents needed to complete the experiment, and followed by a detailed procedure that is supported with a helpful notes section offering tips and tricks of the trade as well as troubleshooting advice. These hallmark features were introduced by series editor Dr. John Walker and constitute the key ingredient in each and every volume of the *Methods in Molecular Biology* series. Tested and trusted, comprehensive and reliable, all protocols from the series are indexed in PubMed.

Rhinovirus

Methods and Protocols

Edited by

Umadevi Sajjan

Lewis Katz School of Medicine, Temple University, Philadelphia, PA, USA

Humana Press

Editor
Umadevi Sajjan
Lewis Katz School of Medicine
Temple University
Philadelphia, PA, USA

ISSN 1064-3745 ISSN 1940-6029 (electronic)
Methods in Molecular Biology
ISBN 978-1-0716-4412-6 ISBN 978-1-0716-4410-2 (eBook)
https://doi.org/10.1007/978-1-0716-4410-2

This Humana imprint is published by the registered company Springer Science+Business Media, LLC, part of Springer Nature.
The registered company address is: 1 New York Plaza, New York, NY 10004, U.S.A.

Preface

Rhinovirus (RV) infections are associated with 70% of the common colds. Infections with RV usually cause mild upper respiratory symptoms such as runny nose, sore throat, stuffiness and sometimes slightly increased body temperature, which is usually self-limited. Airway epithelial cells are the primary target for RV infection. RV does not cause excessive epithelial damage, but induces expression of potent chemoattractants, which recruit polymorphonuclear cells (PMNs). The upper respiratory symptoms usually coincide with the infiltration of PMNs. In infants, elderly and immunocompromised patients, it causes severe respiratory disease sometimes requiring hospitalization. Infants who experience RV-induced wheezing and develop respiratory allergies are at high risk for development of childhood asthma. In these patients, RV infections continue to be a major cause of acute wheezing illness. In patients with chronic lung diseases, such as asthma, cystic fibrosis and chronic obstructive pulmonary disease, RV infections are associated with exacerbations. Experimental infection with RV in asthma and COPD patients causes persistent and severe lung inflammation. Following experimental infection, RV was detected in the subepithelium and macrophages. In addition, a new species RV-C has been recognized to be associated with disease severity, particularly in patients with asthma. These findings have increased our interest in understanding the molecular mechanisms of RV-induced pathogenesis and RV biology. These studies have led to refinement of existing and development of new laboratory techniques, validated mouse models, new and rapid methods to detect RV in clinical samples. To further our knowledge and understanding of RV pathogenesis, it is necessary to share the current methodologies.

There are more than 100 serotypes of RVs. Based on sequence similarities, RV types are classified into three species. The A and B species were first identified decades ago, while RV-C was first described in 2006. V-As include 80 serotypes, RV-Bs include 32 serotypes, and the recently found RV-C species contains at least 57 serotypes. Approximately 89 serotypes of RV-A and -B species belong to the major group and bind to human ICAM-1, thus showing the species specificity. The minor group RVs, which consist of at least 12 serotypes of RV-A, bind to the low-density lipoprotein receptor (LDLR) family with no species specificity. RV-C binds to cadherin 3, a member of the cadherin family of transmembrane proteins. Although monolayer cultures of HeLa cells and airway epithelial cell lines have provided a basic understanding of RV biology, development of mucociliary-differentiated airway epithelial cell cultures established from airway basal cells of normal subjects, COPD and asthma patients has given insights into RV-induced severe disease in patients with chronic lung disease. Unlike cell lines, the mucociliary-differentiated cultures express receptors for all three species of RV and can be used for comparing the outcomes of infection. Majority of in vivo studies are conducted with minor group RV that bind to LDLR due to species specificity. A humanized ICAM-1 mouse has also been developed to examine the immune responses induced by major group RV. These in vivo models have advanced our understanding of the immune responses to RV. The baby mouse model of RV infection has invaluable insights into mechanisms underlying development of childhood asthma.

Methods for isolation of RV have come a long way and now it is possible to obtain relatively pure and high-titer virus by ultrafiltration. This method can be used for purification of all three species of RV. The ability to obtain high titer virus that could be used in vitro and in vivo and the validated models will help us to understand the molecular mechanisms by which RV causes severe lower respiratory tract disease in patients with COPD and asthma.

This volume describes methods to detect RV in clinical samples, propagation and purification of virus, in vivo and in vitro model systems, and the newer molecular tools that are useful for studying the RV infection and pathogenesis. The approaches provided here have led to a greater of understanding of RV pathogenesis in COPD, childhood asthma development and protective innate immunity. However, there is much to learn about RV infection in order to develop therapies to treat asthma and COPD exacerbations, prevent development of asthma and treat common colds.

Philadelphia, PA, USA ***Umadevi Sajjan***

Contents

Preface .... *v*
Contributors .... *ix*

1 Detection of Rhinovirus in Clinical Samples by PCR 1
Mohsen Tabasi

2 Laboratory Protocol for Propagation and Purification of Rhinovirus A and B Suitable for In Vitro and In Vivo Infection 9
Haleh Ganjian and Umadevi Sajjan

3 Method to Generate High-Titer Rhinovirus C Suitable for In Vitro and In Vivo Studies 21
Umadevi Sajjan

4 Quantification of Infectious Rhinovirus A and B Serotypes by Plaque Assay ... 31
Mohsen Tabasi, Haleh Ganjian, and Umadevi Sajjan

5 Quantifying Rhinovirus Genomic and Negative-Strand RNA by RT-PCR..... 39
Shahina Wiehler, Michelle E. Love, and David Proud

6 Determination of Binding and Endocytosis of Rhinovirus by Flow Cytometry 51
Umadevi Sajjan

7 Assessment of Viral Replication in Rhinovirus-Infected Airway Epithelial Cells 65
Michelle E. Love, Shahina Wiehler, and David Proud

8 Analysis of Adherence Junctions in Rhinovirus-Infected Airway Epithelial Cells 77
Kevin Looi, Liisa M. Hirvonen, and Anthony Kicic

9 Culturing of Airway Stem Cells Obtained from COPD Patients to Assess the Effects of Rhinovirus Infection 97
Mohsen Tabasi, Tyler Markward, and Umadevi Sajjan

10 Investigation of Differentiated Nasal Epithelial Responses to Infection with Clinical Isolates of *Rhinovirus* A and C 113
Rebecca L. Watkinson, Yury A. Bochkov, James E. Gern, Thomas Iosifidis, Kevin Looi, Ingrid A. Laing, and Anthony Kicic

11 In Vivo Model to Assess the Nasal Infection by Minor Group Rhinovirus..... 141
Umadevi Sajjan

12 Identification and Analysis of Type 2 Innate Lymphoid Cells in Rhinovirus-Infected Mouse Model of Asthma........ 153
Charu Rajput

13 Assessment of Rhinovirus Infection in a Mouse Model of COPD 165
Krist H. Antunes, Millie M. Jackson, Kyle T. Mincham, Robert J. Snelgrove, and Aran Singanayagam

14 Infection of Immature Mice with Rhinovirus for the Study of Asthma Pathogenesis 173
Mingyuan Han and Marc Hershenson

15 In Vitro Model to Test Therapeutic Agents Against Rhinovirus Infection. 185
Elizabeth McCluskey and Umadevi Sajjan

Index *193*

Contributors

KRIST H. ANTUNES • *Laboratory of Clinical and Experimental Immunology, Pontifical Catholic University of Rio Grande do Sul, Porto Alegre, Brazil*

YURY A. BOCHKOV • *Department of Paediatrics, School of Medicine and Public Health, University of Wisconsin, Madison, WI, USA*

HALEH GANJIAN • *Centre for Inflammation and Lung Research, Lewis Katz Medical School, Temple University, Philadelphia, PA, USA*

JAMES E. GERN • *Department of Paediatrics, School of Medicine and Public Health, University of Wisconsin, Madison, WI, USA*

MINGYUAN HAN • *Department of Pediatrics, University of Michigan Medical School, Ann Arbor, MI, USA*

MARC HERSHENSON • *Department of Pediatrics, University of Michigan Medical School, Ann Arbor, MI, USA; Department of Molecular and Integrative Physiology, University of Michigan Medical School, Ann Arbor, MI, USA*

LIISA M. HIRVONEN • *Centre for Microscopy, Characterisation and Analysis (CMCA), University of Western Australia, Crawley, WA, Australia*

THOMAS IOSIFIDIS • *Division of Paediatrics, School of Medicine, The University of Western Australia, Crawley, WA, Australia; Wal-Yan Respiratory Research Centre, The Kids Research Institute Australia, Nedlands, WA, Australia; School of Population Health, Curtin University, Bentley, WA, Australia; Centre for Cell Therapy and Regenerative Medicine, The University of Western Australia, Crawley, WA, Australia*

MILLIE M. JACKSON • *Department of Infectious Disease, Imperial College London, London, UK*

ANTHONY KICIC • *Wal-yan Respiratory Research Centre, The Kids Research Institute Australia, Nedlands, WA, Australia; School of Public Health, Curtin University, Bentley, WA, Australia; Faculty of Health and Medical Science, University of Western Australia, Crawley, WA, Australia; Department of Respiratory and Sleep Medicine, Perth Children's Hospital, Nedlands, WA, Australia; Centre for Cell Therapy and Regenerative Medicine, The University of Western Australia, Crawley, WA, Australia*

INGRID A. LAING • *Division of Paediatrics, School of Medicine, The University of Western Australia, Crawley, WA, Australia; Wal-Yan Respiratory Research Centre, The Kids Research Institute Australia, Nedlands, WA, Australia; Division of Cardiovascular and Respiratory Sciences, School of Biomedical Sciences, University of Western Australia, Crawley, WA, Australia*

KEVIN LOOI • *Division of Paediatrics, School of Medicine, The University of Western Australia, Crawley, WA, Australia; Wal-Yan Respiratory Research Centre, The Kids Research Institute Australia, Nedlands, WA, Australia; School of Population Health, Curtin University, Bentley, WA, Australia*

MICHELLE E. LOVE • *Department of Physiology and Pharmacology, and Snyder Institute for Chronic Diseases, Cumming School of Medicine, University of Calgary, Calgary, AB, Canada*

TYLER MARKWARD • *Centre for Inflammation and Lung Research, Lewis Katz Medical School, Temple University, Philadelphia, PA, USA*

ELIZABETH MCCLUSKEY • *Centre for Inflammation and Lung Research, Lewis Katz Medical School, Temple University, Philadelphia, PA, USA*

KYLE T. MINCHAM • *National Heart and Lung Institute, Imperial College London, London, UK*

DAVID PROUD • *Department of Physiology and Pharmacology, and Snyder Institute for Chronic Diseases, Cumming School of Medicine, University of Calgary, Calgary, AB, Canada*

CHARU RAJPUT • *Centre for Inflammation and Lung Research, Lewis Katz Medical School, Temple University, Philadelphia, PA, USA*

UMADEVI SAJJAN • *Centre for Inflammation and Lung Research, Lewis Katz Medical School, Temple University, Philadelphia, PA, USA; Department of Microbiology, Immunology and Inflammation, Temple University, Philadelphia, PA, USA; Department of Thoracic Medicine and Surgery, Temple University, Philadelphia, PA, USA*

ARAN SINGANAYAGAM • *Department of Infectious Disease, Imperial College London, London, UK; National Heart and Lung Institute, Imperial College London, London, UK*

ROBERT J. SNELGROVE • *National Heart and Lung Institute, Imperial College London, London, UK*

MOHSEN TABASI • *Centre for Inflammation and Lung Research, Lewis Katz Medical School, Temple University, Philadelphia, PA, USA; Department of Microbiology, Immunology and Inflammation, Lewis Katz Medical School, Temple University, Philadelphia, PA, USA; Department of Thoracic Medicine and Surgery, Lewis Katz Medical School, Temple University, Philadelphia, PA, USA*

REBECCA L. WATKINSON • *Division of Paediatrics, School of Medicine, The University of Western Australia, Crawley, WA, Australia; Wal-Yan Respiratory Research Centre, The Kids Research Institute Australia, Nedlands, WA, Australia*

SHAHINA WIEHLER • *Department of Physiology and Pharmacology, and Snyder Institute for Chronic Diseases, Cumming School of Medicine, University of Calgary, Calgary, AB, Canada*

Chapter 1

Detection of Rhinovirus in Clinical Samples by PCR

Mohsen Tabasi

Abstract

Rhinovirus is a prevalent respiratory pathogen responsible for a significant proportion of upper and lower respiratory tract infections. Its ability to cause a range of illnesses, from mild common cold symptoms to more severe respiratory diseases, underscores the importance of accurate and timely detection. Detecting rhinovirus in clinical samples is an important diagnostic process for identifying and diagnosing respiratory infections caused by this common virus. This chapter of the book provides a comprehensive overview of the methodologies and techniques employed in the detection of rhinovirus in clinical samples.

Key words Detection, Diagnosis, Rhinovirus, Real-time PCR

1 Introduction

Human rhinoviruses (RV) are a group of small, non-enveloped viruses that belong to the family Picornaviridae, genus *Enterovirus*. RVs are single-stranded, positive-sense RNA viruses with an icosahedral symmetrical capsid [1]. The genome is approximately 7200 bp and encodes four structural proteins, VP1, VP2, VP3, and VP4, which make up the viral capsid, and seven non-structural proteins, 2A, 2B, 2C, 3B, 3C, and 3D, which participate in the RV genome replication and polypeptide processing [2].

RVs exhibit a remarkable degree of genetic diversity. Based on sequence variation, a phylogenic tree was generated, which classified RV into three different species: RV-A, RV-B, and RV-C [3]. This diversity contributes to the wide range of clinical presentations, from common colds to severe respiratory tract infections. The traditional serological method is challenging and cumbersome given the existence of more than 100 serotypes. To determine the relationship between the specific strains of RV and the illnesses, nested reverse transcription (RT)-PCR and multiplex PCR and real-time PCR [4–7] methods have been developed. These methods are more sensitive, faster, and less laborious. For example,

Umadevi Sajjan (ed.), *Rhinovirus: Methods and Protocols*, Methods in Molecular Biology, vol. 2903,
https://doi.org/10.1007/978-1-0716-4410-2_1,

one-step real-time PCR is 100 to 1000-fold more sensitive than culture-based assays and highly reproducible. This assay can be completed within 5 h. In this chapter, we will provide detailed methods for collecting and processing of samples and real-time PCR methods for the detection of RV in clinical samples. These methods can be used for the detection of RV in nasal swabs, nasal lavage, and BAL lavage and will identify all three groups of RV but will not differentiate between the three species.

2 Materials

2.1 Clinical Samples, Transport Medium, and Storage (See Note 1)

1. UTM with flocked swabs (Copan Cat # 360C/305C).
2. Sterile saline.
3. Sterile tubes.
4. Nasopharyngeal swab in viral transport medium.
5. Nasopharyngeal aspirate in viral transport medium.

2.2 Total RNA Isolation

1. Quick-RNA™ Viral kit (Zymo research) or any other viral RNA extraction kit (*see* **Note 1**).
2. Molecular biology grade absolute alcohol.
3. Carrier RNA (ThermoFisher Cat# 4382878).
4. DNase and RNase-free tubes 1.5 mL microcentrifuge tubes.
5. RNase-free filter pipette tips.
6. Microcentrifuge.
7. Nanodrop.

2.3 PCR Kits and Other Accessories

1. ViroReal® kit Rhinovirus (A, B, C) (ingenetix) detects rhinovirus A/B/C.
2. Quant studio 7 (ThermoFisher) or any other real-time PCR machine that can detect FAM and Cy5.
3. 96-Well PCR plate
4. Optical plate sealing adhesive film.
5. RNase-free filter tips.

3 Methods

3.1 Sample Preparation

1. All samples must be collected in sterile tubes in the clinic and should be transported to the laboratory within 24 h (*see* **Note 2**).
2. Two types of samples can be used for RV detection: nasopharyngeal swabs and nasopharyngeal aspirates. The latter requires

specialized equipment and should be collected by licensed physicians according to local safety protocol.

3. Nasal swabs should be transported in virus transport medium. The swabs are squeezed against the wall of the tubes and removed. The sample should be immediately mixed with an equal volume of 2× DNA/RNA Shield (provided in the viral RNA isolation kit) and stored at −80 °C in aliquots.
4. Nasopharyngeal aspirates should be thoroughly mixed with an equal volume of 2× DNA/RNA Shield and stored at 80 °C in aliquots.

3.2 Extraction of Viral RNA

1. The method summarizes a modified version of the manufacturer's instructions to isolate Viral RNA suitable for RV detection using the ViroReal® kit Rhinovirus A/B/C.
2. Perform all the steps and centrifugation at room temperature. Set the microcentrifuge speed at 10.000–16,000× *g*.
3. Add 250 μL of β-mercaptoethanol to 50 mL of Viral RNA Buffer.
4. Add 24 mL of 100% (absolute) ethanol to the 6 mL of Viral Wash Buffer concentrate.
5. Bring all the samples to room temperature before starting RNA extraction. If using a fresh sample, mix one-to-one with 2× DNA/RNA Shield (200 μL of sample with 200 μL of 2× DNA/RNA Shield). Add 1 μL of carrier RNA (*see* **Note 3**).
6. To 400 μL of sample, add 800 μL of Viral RNA Buffer (1:2) and mix well. Spike with 1 μL of RNA IPC Target (internal RNA positive control) from the ViroReal® kit Rhinovirus A/B/C (*see* **Note 4**).
7. Assemble the spin columns by placing the Zymo-Spin™ IC column in a 2 mL collection tube (one column per sample).
8. Transfer the mixture into the assembled spin columns and centrifuge for 2 min (*see* **Note 5**).
9. Transfer the column to a new collection tube. At this step, DNase I treatment can be performed to remove DNA and obtain pure viral RNA (*see* **Note 6**).
10. Add 500 μL of Viral Wash Buffer to the column, centrifuge for 30 s, and discard the flow-through.
11. Repeat **step 10**.
12. Add 500 μL of absolute ethanol to the column and centrifuge for 30 s. Discard the flow-through and centrifuge again for 30 s to remove traces of ethanol.
13. Carefully transfer the column to a new 1.5 mL RNase-free collection tube (*see* **Note 7**).

14. Add 15 μL of RNase/DNase-free water directly to the column matrix and centrifuge for 30 s (*see* **Note 8**).
15. Include a negative sample that only has carrier RNA and spike with 1 μL of RNA IPC (internal RNA positive control) from The ViroReal® kit Rhinovirus A/B/C (*see* **Note 9**) and process this sample similarly to clinical samples. This will be used as a negative control of the RNA in one-step PCR.

3.3 One-Step qPCR for Detecting Rhinovirus A, B, and C

1. The ViroReal® kit Rhinovirus detects RNA of the 5″ UTR of the rhinovirus species A, B, and C. The method described here summarizes the manufacturer's instructions.
2. Use freshly isolated RNA or frozen RNA. Thaw frozen RNA samples on ice and stable on ice for up to 8 h.
3. Preparing master mix. The following table lists the volume of each reagent per reaction. Based on the number of samples, multiply the volume given in Table 1 by the number of samples. Always make the master mix for one extra sample.
4. Preparing PCR mix: Aliquot 15 μL of master mix to each well in a 96-well plate or strip well 0.2 mL thin-walled tubes. Add 5 μL of RNA sample (*see* **Note 9**). Seal the plate with an optically clear adhesive cover.
5. Programming of real-time PCR machine:
    1. Detection channels—FAM-TAMRA for detection of rhinovirus; Cy5-NONE for detection of IPC; ROX passive reference dye.
    2. Temperature and number of cycles (Table 2):
6. Data interpretation: Select the FAM and Cy5 channels to get the Ct values for each sample. The FAM channel is for rhinovirus, and the Cy5 channel is for the RNA IPC target.
7. The amplification curve should be inspected both in log and linear scale and compared with negative controls. Adjust the threshold, if necessary (Table 3).

Table 1
Master mix

Reagents	Volume per reaction (μL)
Nuclease-free water	8.0
RNA reaction mix	5.0
Rhinovirus assay mix	1.0
RNA IPC-3 assay mix	1.0
Total volume master mix	15.0

Table 2
Set up of PCR machine

	Step 1 reverse transcription	Step 2 polymerase activation	Step 3 analysis: quantification and acquisition	
No of cycles	1	1	45	
Temperature	50 °C	95 °C	95 °C	60 °C
Time	15 min	20 s	5 s	1 min

Table 3
below criteria for valid controls

	Ct FAM channel rhinovirus	Ct Cy5 channel RNA IPC target	Interpretation	Notes
Positive control	26–28	Negative	Valid	
Positive control	Negative	Negative	Invalid	10
Positive control	26–28	Positive	Invalid	11
Extraction negative control	Negative	25–28	Valid	
Extraction negative control	Negative	Negative	Invalid	
Extraction negative control	Positive	25–28	Invalid	11
Negative control (optional)	Negative	Negative	Valid	
Negative control (optional)	Positive	Negative	Invalid	12
Negative control (optional)	Negative	Positive	Invalid	12

8. Assessment of clinical samples should be performed after the negative and positive controls are examined and determined to be valid and satisfactory. If the positive and negative controls are not valid, then the clinical samples cannot be interpreted. Please see Table 4 for the interpretation of clinical samples.

4 Notes

1. RNA isolation kit, Zymo Research Viral RNA extraction kit is simple to use and yields highly purified RNA that is suitable for qPCR and nextgen sequencing if needed for molecular typing of the virus.

Table 4
Interpretation of data with clinical samples

	Ct FAM channel rhinovirus	Ct Cy5 Channel RNA IPC target	Interpretation	Notes
Clinical sample	Negative	26–28 (*see* **Note 14**)	Negative	
Clinical sample	Positive	Positive	Positive	
Clinical sample	Positive	Negative (*see* **Note 15**)	Positive	
Clinical sample	Negative	25–28	Valid	**13**

2. Sample analysis within 24 h of the collection is advisable but otherwise can be stored at 2–8 °C.
3. Given that a very small amount of RNA is present in the clinical sample, it is necessary to add carrier RNA to a total of 1 μg.
4. The samples should be spiked with the RNA IPC from the ViroReal kit to exclude false-negative results due to inhibition of reverse transcription real-time PCR downstream of RNA isolation.
5. RNA and DNA bind to the matrix in the column and at this step. At this step, an additional 400 μL of sample can be added to the column if more RNA is needed for the downstream procedure.
6. Treatment with DNase I digests all the DNA to yield pure RNA. This step is optional.
7. Always handle the column at the top. Touching the bottom of the column can degrade the RNA.
8. If highly concentrated RNA is needed, use ≥6 μL elution. The eluted RNA can be used immediately or stored frozen at −80 ° C. RNA concentration can be measured by the Nanodrop method if required.
9. When using higher than 5 μL of RNA sample, reduce the water in the master mix so that the total volume of PCR mix is 20 μL.
10. No virus-specific signal with positive control and with IPC should check the following.
    1. The programming of the temperature profile in the real-time PCR is incorrect.
    2. If the setup of the PCR reaction is incorrect, repeat PCR.
    3. If the RNA IPC target was not added to the samples before RNA extraction and if it was added directly to the PCR mix, use 1 μL of 1:500 diluted RNA IPC.
    4. Make sure the positive control RNA was added to the PCR mix.

11. Virus-specific signal (FAM) in the negative control and negative control of extraction. This is due to contamination with the positive control RNA or sample. Repeat the RT-PCR with new reagents, set up the positive control at the end, and always clean the bench before extraction of RNA from the sample and while setting up the RT-PCR reaction. Always use aerosol pipette tips in all the steps. If the virus-specific signal is observed in the negative control of extraction, repeat RNA extraction and RT-PCR.
12. IPC-specific signals in negative control and positive control indicate contamination with the RNA IPC target. Make sure that the workspace and the instruments are decontaminated at regular intervals.
13. No signal with IPC and no virus-specific signal with the sample indicate that PCR reaction was inhibited. If there are no mistakes during the extraction of RNA, the RNA may be too low for the detection of the virus. Use 6 μL of water to elute the RNA from the column (refer to **Note 8**). Also, one should check the setup of the PCR reaction and RT-PCR conditions.
14. A positive signal in RNA IPC excludes PCR inhibition. However, IPC Ct values should show comparable results among samples. A shift in Ct values indicates a partial inhibition of PCR.
15. High pathogen load in the sample can inhibit RNA IPC target amplification. Dilute the RNA and repeat the PCR.

References

1. Palmenberg AC, Gern JE (2015) Classification and evolution of human rhinoviruses. Methods Mol Biol 1221:1–10
2. Arnold E, Rossmann MG (1990) Analysis of the structure of a common cold virus, human rhinovirus 14, refined at a resolution of 3.0 a. J Mol Biol 211:763–801
3. Palmenberg AC, Spiro D, Kuzmickas R, Wang S, Djikeng A, Rathe JA, Fraser-Liggett CM, Liggett SB (2009) Sequencing and analyses of all known human rhinovirus genomes reveal structure and evolution. Science 324:55–59
4. Andeweg AC, Bestebroer TM, Huybreghs M, Kimman TG, de Jong JC (1999) Improved detection of rhinoviruses in clinical samples by using a newly developed nested reverse transcription-PCR assay. J Clin Microbiol 37: 524–530
5. Silva ER, Watanabe AS, Carraro E, Perosa AH, Granato CF, Bellei NC (2012) Rhinovirus detection using different PCR-based strategies. Braz J Microbiol 43:739–743
6. Feng ZS, Zhao L, Wang J, Qiu FZ, Zhao MC, Wang L, Duan SX, Zhang RQ, Chen C, Qi JJ et al (2018) A multiplex one-tube nested real time RT-PCR assay for simultaneous detection of respiratory syncytial virus, human rhinovirus and human metapneumovirus. Virol J 15:167
7. Do DH, Laus S, Leber A, Marcon MJ, Jordan JA, Martin JM, Wadowsky RM (2010) A one-step, real-time PCR assay for rapid detection of rhinovirus. J Mol Diagn 12:102–108

Chapter 2

Laboratory Protocol for Propagation and Purification of Rhinovirus A and B Suitable for In Vitro and In Vivo Infection

Haleh Ganjian and Umadevi Sajjan

Abstract

H1HeLa cell line has become the most utilized cell culture system for in vitro studies of the rhinovirus life cycle. These cells are also widely used to propagate the rhinovirus to study host responses. Unlike other viruses, high-titer virus is required for studies focusing on understanding the host responses to rhinovirus infection in vivo and in vitro. Therefore, after propagation of rhinovirus, H1HeLa cells should be concentrated and purified. In this chapter, we describe the methods used for the propagation of rhinovirus A and B that are adapted to H1HeLa cells.

Key words H1HeLa cells, Viral purification, Ultracentrifugation

1 Introduction

Human rhinoviruses (RV) are small, non-enveloped viruses with single-stranded, positive-sense RNA. RVs belong to the Picornaviridae family and are divided, based on the phylogeny, into three different species: RV-A, RV-B, and RV-C [1]. There are more than 100 serotypes of RV-A and RV-B and > 50 serotypes of RV-C. RV causes upper respiratory infection, which is associated with common cold symptoms. In addition, RV infections are also linked to acute otitis media and rhinosinusitis, which also coincide with bacterial infections, indicating that RV may increase the risk of acquiring secondary bacterial infections [2]. Furthermore, RV infections are also associated with exacerbations in persons with chronic airway diseases such as chronic obstructive pulmonary disease, asthma, and cystic fibrosis patients [3–6]. Airway epithelial cells are the major target for RVs. All three species of RVs gain entry into host cells by binding to plasma membrane glycoproteins. Based on the receptors that the RV binds to, RV-A and RV-B are classified into major and minor group viruses. Approximately

Umadevi Sajjan (ed.), *Rhinovirus: Methods and Protocols*, Methods in Molecular Biology, vol. 2903,
https://doi.org/10.1007/978-1-0716-4410-2_2,

89 serotypes of RV-A and RV-B are classified under major groups and bind to human ICAM-1 to gain entry into the cells [7]. The rest of the RV-A and RV-B serotypes bind to low-density lipoproteins (LDL) and LDL-like receptors, and these viruses are classified under minor group viruses. RV-C binds to human CDHR3, a member of the cadherin family of transmembrane proteins [8].

The prototype strains of RV-A and RV-B that are commonly used in the laboratory are available from ATCC and can be propagated in the laboratory using H1HeLa cells. RV-C cells can be propagated in mucociliary-differentiated human tracheobronchial epithelial cell cultures but to a very low titer. The HeLa cell line, which is the first immortal cell line, has been extensively used by many laboratories to study cellular and molecular functions of the cells. Due to different cell culture conditions, various HeLa cell lines have evolved over 80 years. A strain known as H1HeLa was found to be highly permissive to RV-A and RV-B and has become the standard cell line to propagate RV and investigate the RV lifecycle, such as virion receptor interactions, viral entry, and viral genome replication and assembly of virus and host responses.

RV-A and RV-B readily infect H1HeLa cells and replicate efficiently in these cells. However, compared to other virulent viruses, or closely related enteroviruses, RVs have significantly lower progeny virus yields. For investigation on RV-stimulated inflammatory and antiviral responses, it is essential to use appropriate cell culture and in vivo models. But such studies require a high-titer virus that is free of cellular components. In previous studies, H1HeLa cells grown in suspension cultures were used to generate concentrated virus [9]. In this method, isolated progeny virus has to be purified by sucrose cushion gradient and gradient centrifugation, and the final yield was very low. The virus used by this method is also not suitable for infecting mice, because even after the removal of sucrose by dialysis, the virus preparation caused excessive inflammation in mice. Moreover, not all the laboratories are equipped with preparative ultracentrifuge. Here we describe a simple method to generate a concentrated virus which is essentially free of cellular components. In addition, the RV prepared by this method was found to be suitable for in vivo experiments [10–12]. The method was developed in our laboratory 20 years ago and is routinely used to generate high-titer virus suitable for both in vivo and in vitro studies.

The method described here entails ultrafiltration of the spent medium from cell cultures infected with RV or sham-infected cultures. Ultrafiltration is a combined method used to concentrate and dialyze the samples at the same time. Ultrafiltration uses a membrane with varying pore size to remove solutes with molecular weight 2 kDA to <100 kDa. Virions are bigger and do not pass through the 100 kDa cutoff membrane. In addition, serum proteins, other media components, and most of the cellular proteins have molecular weight less than 100 kDa. Therefore, we recommend using an ultrafiltration membrane with 100 kDa cutoff to remove all the proteins and concentrate the virus at the same time.

2 Materials

1. H1Hela cells stock (ATCC CRL-1958) (*see* **Note 1**).
2. Rhinovirus stocks RV16 (ATCC VR-283), RV14 (ATCC VR-284), RV1B (ATCC VR-1648) (*see* **Note 2**).
3. Fetal bovine serum.
4. DMEM-high glucose (Gibco, 11965092 or equivalent).
5. Complete medium (DMEM, 1% L-Glutamine, 1% Pen/Strep, 10% Fetal bovine serum).
6. Low serum medium (DMEM, 1% L-Glutamine, 1% Pen/-Strep, 1 or 3% Fetal bovine serum).
7. Infection medium (DMEM, 1% L-Glutamine, 1% Pen/Strep).
8. Cell storage medium (Serum-free medium, 10% DMSO, 10% Fetal bovine serum).
9. Trypsin/EDTA: 0.25% (w/v) trypsin/0.02% (w/v) EDTA (Gibco 25200056 or equivalent).
10. Sterile cell culture-grade PBS without $CaCl_2$ and $MgCl_2$.
11. Endotoxin-free sterile PBS with $CaCl_2$ and $MgCl_2$.
12. Cell culture incubator set at 37 °C.
13. Cell culture incubator set at 33 °C.
14. Liquid nitrogen tank.
15. 100 mm × 15 mm tissue-culture-treated plates
16. 150 mm × 25 mm tissue-culture-treated plates
17. Biosafety Level 2 cell culture hood.
18. A benchtop refrigerated centrifuge.
19. Millipore Amicon Stirred Ultrafiltration Cell (Cat# UFSC40001) (Fig. 1).
20. 100 kDa cutoff ultrafiltration membranes (Millipore Sigma cat#PLHK07610)
21. Filter units with 0.45 cutoff membrane.
22. Glass filters to fit the filter units.
23. Sterile 2-mL cryovials.
24. Nitrogen gas tank with regulator.
25. Magnetic stirrer.
26. Access to cold room.

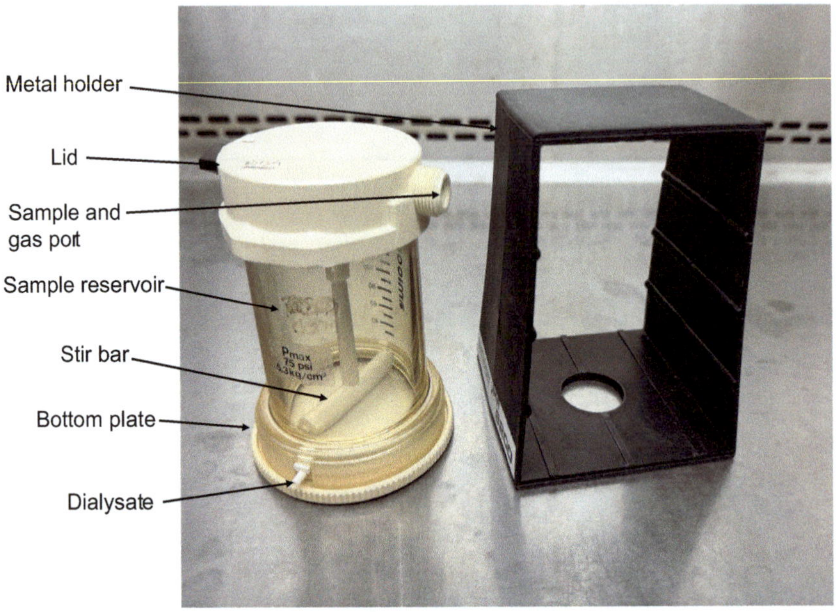

Fig. 1 Ultrafiltration unit: The ultrafiltration unit has two main components. The ultrafiltration cell and the metal holder to place the ultrafiltration cell. The latter has for main components. Sample reservoir, top lid with gas, and sample port, suspended stir bar and the bottom plate. There are two gaskets, one in the lid and one on the bottom plate. The top lid snap closure and the bottom plate has threads to fit it to the ultrafiltration cell

3 Methods

3.1 Preparation of H1HeLa Cell Stocks

1. Warm up complete medium in a 37 °C water bath.
2. Aliquot 10 mL of warm medium into 15 mL sterile conical tube in a cell culture hood.
3. Thaw a frozen vial of H1HeLa cells (*see* **Note 1**) in a 37 °C water bath for 1 min. Make sure that the contents in the vial are not completely thawed.
4. Sterilize the outside of the vial with 70% ethanol and transfer the vial to the cell culture hood.
5. Transfer cells from the vial to a 15 mL centrifuge tube containing 10 mL of warm medium. Invert gently two times to mix the content.
6. Centrifuge for 5 min at 500× *g*, 4 °C, and remove supernatant by aspiration.
7. Resuspend the cell pellet in 1 mL of complete medium and transfer it to a 10-cm cell culture dish containing 10 mL of complete medium. Gently rock the dish to evenly distribute the cells.

8. Incubate the cell culture dish in a cell culture incubator at 37 °C. Change the medium every 2 days.
9. When the cells reach 70–80% confluency, aspirate the medium and rinse the plate two times with 10 mL PBS without $CaCl_2$ and $MgCl_2$.
10. Add 3 mL of trypsin/EDTA and place it in the incubator for up to 2 min.
11. Tap the plate gently against the palm to release the adherent cells.
12. Add 10 mL of complete medium and transfer cells to a sterile 50-mL centrifuge tube.
13. Add 10 mL PBS to the plate and transfer it to a tube containing the cells.
14. Centrifuge for 5 min at 500× *g*, 4 °C, and remove supernatant by aspiration.
15. Resuspend the cell pellet in 5 mL of the complete medium by pipetting up and down.
16. Count the cells using a cell counter or hemacytometer and suspend the cells in the complete medium to adjust the cell density to $1–3 \times 10^6$ cells/mL.
17. Plate cells in three 10 cm dishes (5×10^5 cells/dish), which will be used in Subheading 3.2.
18. For cryopreservation of H1HeLa cells, adjust the cell density to $1–2 \times 10^6$ cells/mL and add DMSO to 10% to the cell suspension. Aliquot 1 mL of cell suspension into cryovials and place it in a chilled freezer box at −80 °C.
19. Transfer cryovials after 24 h into the liquid nitrogen tank for long-term storage.

3.2 Preparation of Viral Seeding Stocks

1. Culture H1HeLa cells in 10-cm dishes as described in Subheading 3.1.
2. Incubate in a cell culture incubator at 37 °C until cells become 90% confluent.
3. Dilute RV (*see* **Note 2**) in the infection medium so that when 3 mL of virus is added, the multiplicity of infection (MOI) is 1–3 pfu/cell.
4. Aspirate media from the culture plate.
5. Add 3 mL of diluted virus suspension to the monolayer cells and incubate for 90 min in a cell culture incubator at 37 °C, gently rock the plate every 15 min so that the infection medium covers the cell monolayer. Do not let the cell monolayer dry.
6. Add 7 mL of complete medium and incubate at 33 °C for another 24 h (*see* **Note 3**).

7. Change the medium with complete medium and continue to incubate the cells for 24–48 h at 33 °C.
8. At this time, the majority of the cells will be cytopathic and will float. Gently pipette the medium up and down to release the cells from the plate and collect the medium along with the cells.
9. Subject the contents of the plates to two freeze-thaw cycles (freezing at −80 °C for 30 min followed by incubation at 37 °C to thaw the cells) to release all the intracellular virus.
10. Centrifuge at 500× *g* for 10 min at 4 °C to pellet the cell debris.
11. Store the supernatants as 0.5 mL aliquots in sterile microcentrifuge tubes and store them at −80 °C. This is the seeding stock to propagate the virus for experiments. Never passage the seeding virus because with each passage, the viral titer will reduce, enriching the cellular components, which can also cause cytopathic effect.

3.3 Propagation of Rhinovirus

3.3.1 Day 1

1. Culture H1HeLa cells in twenty 15-cm cell culture dishes using complete medium until the cells reach 80% confluency.
2. Infect ten plates with rhinovirus seeding stock. For another ten plates, add only the infection medium without the virus.
3. For each plate, dilute 40 μl of viral seeding stock (1×10^8 pfu/mL) in 5 mL of infection medium.
4. Aspirate the medium from cell culture dishes with H1HeLa cells.
5. Add 5 mL of infection medium to each plate (please note that virus-containing infection medium should be added only to ten plates).
6. Incubate at 37 °C for 60 min and slowly rock the plates every 15 min.
7. Add 20 mL of complete medium to each plate. (Do not remove the infection medium from the plate).
8. Incubate for 24 h at 33 °C.

3.3.2 Day 2

1. Change the medium with low serum-containing medium (*see* **Note 4**). Continue incubation at 33 °C.

3.3.3 Days 4 and 5

1. Check plates under a microscope daily for cytopathic effects. This will take 2–3 days, when the cells become rounded and some cells detach from the plate partially (*see* **Note 5**).
2. Collect the spent medium along with floating cells and transfer it to 50 mL sterile centrifuge tubes.
3. Store the tubes at −80 °C until purification. At this stage the virus can be stored for up to 1 month.

3.4 Purification and Concentration of Rhinovirus by Ultrafiltration

1. Loosely close the bottom plate of the ultrafiltration unit, wrap the ultrafiltration unit in aluminum foil, and sterilize the ultrafiltration unit by autoclaving in the liquid cycle. Do not sterilize the membrane in the autoclave.
2. All the steps except for centrifugation and ultrafiltration should be performed in the cell culture hood to maintain the sterility of the virus stock.
3. On the day of purification, thaw the spent medium from sham or virus-infected cells in a water bath at room temperature. (Loosen the caps of the 50 mL tubes to prevent cracking of the tubes).
4. Wipe the outside of the tubes with 70% alcohol and centrifuge at 2000× *g* for 30 min at 4 °C.
5. Collect the supernatant in fresh 50 mL tubes.
6. Discard the cell debris as biohazard waste, because it will contain the infectious virus.
7. While centrifuging the spent medium, prepare the filter unit. Place the glass fiber prefilter on top of the 0.45 μM filter of the filter unit and wet it with sterile PBS. Connect the filter unit to the vacuum. Using a prefilter will prevent clogging of the membrane of the filter unit.
8. Filter the supernatant through the prepared 0.45 filter unit in the cell culture hood. Store the filtrate on ice.
9. Sterilization of ultrafiltration membrane: Immerse 100 kDa cutoff ultrafiltration membrane in a sterile cell culture dish containing 70% alcohol for 15 min.
10. Transfer the membrane to a new plate containing sterile distilled water and soak for 5 min. Repeat this washing step two more times using fresh 20 mL sterile distilled water each time.
11. Transfer the membrane to the bottom plate of the ultrafiltration unit and assemble the ultrafiltration unit as shown in Fig. 2.
12. Add 300 mL of PBS to the ultrafiltration unit. This can be done in two ways. The lid on the top of the filtration cell is snap closed. Take out the lid carefully, leaving the magnetic bar inside the cell. Add the buffer to the cell. The second method is to use a 50 mL sterile syringe attached to a sterile tubing. Fill the syringe, insert the tubing through the sample port, and deliver the sample or buffer to the ultrafiltration cell. This method is preferred to prevent contamination while adding the buffer to the sample. Connect the inlet line to a regulated gas pressure source in a cold room. Use nitrogen gas for pressurizing the cell (Fig. 3) (*see* **Note 6**).
13. Collect the dialyzate from the ultrafiltration unit and discard it.

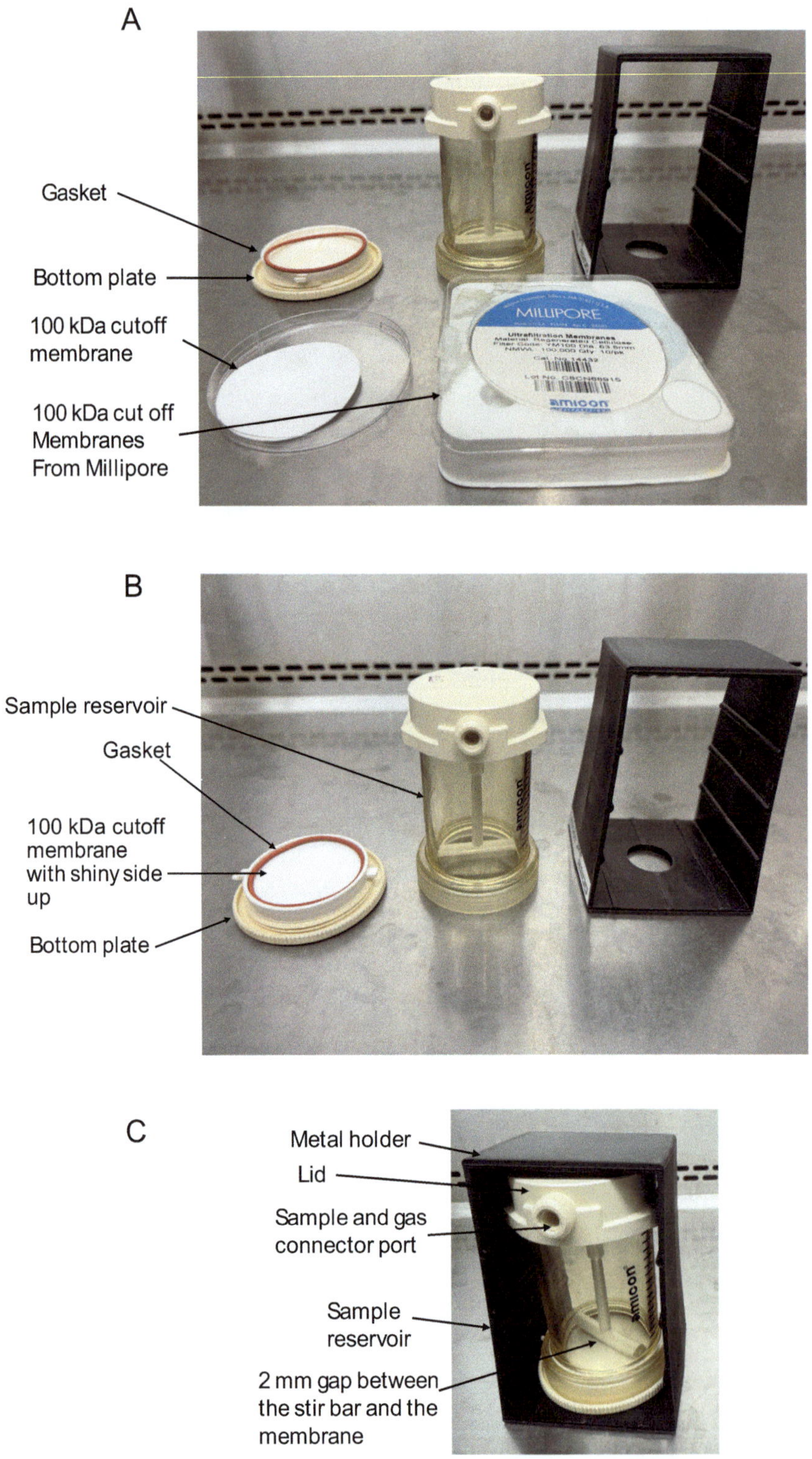

Fig. 2 (**a**): Ultrafiltration unit with membrane: Always handle the membrane with sterile, blunt-ended forceps to prevent damage to the membrane. Do not handle the membrane with bare or gloved hands. Sterilize the membrane in 70% alcohol and rinse with sterile distilled water. Always keep the shiny side of the membrane facing down while sterilizing and washing. (**b**): Assembly of ultrafiltration unit: Remove the gasket from the

14. Repeat this step two more times with fresh 300 mL PBS.
15. Add 300 mL viral supernatant into the ultrafiltration device.
16. Place the unit on the magnetic stirrer, turn on the stirrer to low speed to mix the contents in the ultrafiltration unit, and adjust the stirring rate to very slow.
17. Initially apply low pressure, that is 10–20 Psi, and as the flow rate of the effluent reduces to less than 0.5 mL/min, slowly increase the pressure step-wise. But never exceed 75 Psi (*see* **Note 7**).
18. Wait until the volume decreases to 10–20 mL.
19. Add 300 mL of endotoxin-free PBS, stir at a very slow rate, and apply the pressure to reduce the volume to 10–20 mL.
20. Repeat **step 19** two more times to efficiently dialyze and concentrate the virus.
21. Collect the final concentrate (10 mL) and store it in 0.5 mL aliquots at −80 °C (*see* **Notes 8** and **9**).

This method will yield a partially purified virus that is free of cellular material such as RNA, DNA, cytokines, growth factors, proteases, RNases, DNases, and serum proteins. This partially purified virus is viable, infects airway epithelial cells in vitro and mouse airways in vivo efficiently, and stimulates pro-inflammatory and antiviral responses [13, 14].

4 Notes

1. H1HeLa cells must be tested for mycoplasma contamination (the mycoplasma detection kit can be purchased from Sigma or other suppliers). Sham generated from mycoplasma-contaminated cells will stimulate pro-inflammatory responses in the cells, which is indistinguishable from RV infection. If the cells are contaminated with mycoplasma, the cells should be cured by using a mycoplasma elimination kit (Sigma Aldrich kit

Fig. 2 (continued) bottom plate with the sterile forceps. Transfer the sterile membrane onto the bottom plate with the shiny surface of the membrane facing up with forceps, ensuring the filter fits on the bottom plate. Place the gasket carefully on top of the membrane with forceps and gently push the membrane so that the gasket is fitted on top of the membrane snugly with no bulging. Screw in the reservoir + the lid to the bottom plate. (**c**): Assembled ultrafiltration unit: Assemble the ultrafiltration cell and slide it into the metal holder. Make sure that the stir bar is not touching the membrane surface. There should be a minimum 2 mm gap between the stir bar and the membrane. If the gap is not maintained, the magnetic bar will damage the membrane while stirring. At the top of the reservoir there is a groove where the rod attached to the magnetic bar is fixed. The placement of this rod can be adjusted so that the minimum gap between the membrane and magnetic bar is maintained. This adjustment should be made prior to sterilizing the ultrafiltration cell

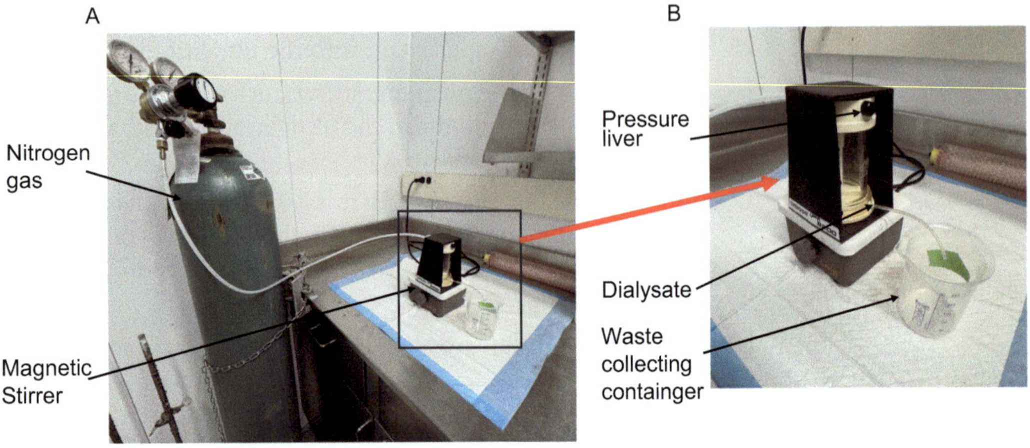

Fig. 3 Connection of ultrafiltration unit to the pressure source: (**a**) Add PBS or sample to the reservoir of the assembled ultrafiltration unit, transfer it to the cold room, and place it on the magnetic stirrer. Connect the unit to the nitrogen gas cylinder. Apply the pressure to 5–10 PSI. Turn the pressure liver anticlockwise so that now it is perpendicular to the ultrafiltration unit. At this time the ultrafiltration cell is closed, and the pressure will be applied to the cell. The lid of the ultrafiltration cell will pop and is held tight by the metal holder. Start the stirrer and set it to low speed. The dialysate that is less than <100 kDa will flow through, which is collected in a waste container. (**b**) is an enlarged image of the area marked in (**a**)

Cat#CUL001B). The cells should be tested for mycoplasma routinely.

2. Some RV stocks obtained from ATCC will have mycoplasma contamination. The mycoplasma from the viral stocks can be removed by treatment with ether. Add 100 μl of ether to 300 μl of viral stock at 4 °C. Vortex for 1 minute, centrifuge at 10,000 g for 5 min. Remove and dilute supernatant to 2 mL with fresh complete media, and infect H1HeLa cells immediately. The RV-infected cells should be tested for mycoplasma.
3. RV replication occurs better at 33 °C than at 37 °C. To obtain high-titer virus, it is important to incubate cells at 33 °C for generating either viral seeding stocks or viral stocks for experiments.
4. A 3% serum-containing medium will yield a higher titer virus. However, the virus is not suitable for in vivo studies. Therefore, we recommend 1% serum-containing medium if the virus is to be used for in vivo infection.
5. Do not wait until all cells are completely detached from the plate. This will increase cellular components and decrease the viral yield.
6. Always use inert gas such as nitrogen to pressurize the ultrafiltration cell. Using compressed air can cause large pH shifts due to the dissolution of carbon dioxide, which will drastically reduce the viral yield.

7. In the beginning, the flow rate of the effluent will be 2–5 mL per minute, and it reduces as the viral supernatant is concentrated in the ultrafiltration unit.
8. Concentrated virus appears as a turbid solution, and this is common because the virus precipitates out of the solution and can be suspended by vortexing or pipetting up and down gently before use.
9. Concentrating 25 mL of supernatant (from one 15 cm plate) to a final volume of 1 mL will yield 3–5 × 10^8 pfu/mL.

References

1. Palmenberg AC, Gern JE (2015) Classification and evolution of human rhinoviruses. Methods Mol Biol 1221:1–10
2. Jacobs SE, Lamson DM, St George K, Walsh TJ (2013) Human rhinoviruses. Clin Microbiol Rev 26:135–162
3. Makela MJ, Puhakka T, Ruuskanen O, Leinonen M, Saikku P, Kimpimaki M, Blomqvist S, Hyypia T, Arstila P (1998) Viruses and bacteria in the etiology of the common cold. J Clin Microbiol 36:539–542
4. Lee WM, Lemanske RF Jr, Evans MD, Vang F, Pappas T, Gangnon R, Jackson DJ, Gern JE (2012) Human rhinovirus species and season of infection determine illness severity. Am J Respir Crit Care Med 186:886–891
5. Etherington C, Naseer R, Conway SP, Whitaker P, Denton M, Peckham DG (2014) The role of respiratory viruses in adult patients with cystic fibrosis receiving intravenous antibiotics for a pulmonary exacerbation. J Cyst Fibros 13:49–55
6. George SN, Garcha DS, Mackay AJ, Patel AR, Singh R, Sapsford RJ, Donaldson GC, Wedzicha JA (2014) Human rhinovirus infection during naturally occurring COPD exacerbations. Eur Respir J 44:87–96
7. Greve JM, Davis G, Meyer AM, Forte CP, Yost SC, Marlor CW, Kamarck ME, McClelland A (1989) The major human rhinovirus receptor is ICAM-1. Cell 56:839–847
8. Bochkov YA, Watters K, Ashraf S, Griggs TF, Devries MK, Jackson DJ, Palmenberg AC, Gern JE (2015) Cadherin-related family member 3, a childhood asthma susceptibility gene product, mediates rhinovirus C binding and replication. Proc Natl Acad Sci USA 112: 5485–5490
9. Lee WM, Chen Y, Wang W, Mosser A (2015) Growth of human rhinovirus in H1-HeLa cell suspension culture and purification of virions. Methods Mol Biol 1221:49–61
10. Newcomb DC, Sajjan US, Nagarkar DR, Wang Q, Nanua S, Zhou Y, McHenry CL, Hennrick KT, Tsai WC, Bentley JK et al (2008) Human rhinovirus 1B exposure induces phosphatidylinositol 3-kinase-dependent airway inflammation in mice. Am J Respir Crit Care Med 177:1111–1121
11. Sajjan U, Ganesan S, Comstock AT, Shim J, Wang Q, Nagarkar DR, Zhao Y, Goldsmith AM, Sonstein J, Linn MJ et al (2009) Elastase- and LPS-exposed mice display altered responses to rhinovirus infection. Am J Physiol Lung Cell Mol Physiol 297:L931–L944
12. Ganesan S, Faris A, Chattoraj S, Comstock A, Hershenson M, Sajjan U (2011) Quercetin improves lung function in rhinovirus-infected mice with a COPD phenotype. Am J Respir Crit Care Med 183:A4581
13. Newcomb DC, Sajjan U, Nanua S, Jia Y, Goldsmith AM, Bentley JK, Hershenson MB (2005) Phosphatidylinositol 3-kinase is required for rhinovirus-induced airway epithelial cell interleukin-8 expression. J Biol Chem 280: 36952–36961
14. Schneider D, Ganesan S, Comstock AT, Meldrum CA, Mahidhara R, Goldsmith AM, Curtis JL, Martinez FJ, Hershenson MB, Sajjan U (2010) Increased cytokine response of rhinovirus-infected airway epithelial cells in chronic obstructive pulmonary disease. Am J Respir Crit Care Med 182:332–340

Chapter 3

Method to Generate High-Titer Rhinovirus C Suitable for In Vitro and In Vivo Studies

Umadevi Sajjan

Abstract

Rhinovirus (RV)-C, discovered in 2006, binds to human cadherin-related family member 3 expressed on ciliated cells. RV-C is the cause of severe respiratory illness in children with asthma. Unlike rhinovirus-A and B, very little is known about the RV-C biology or pathogenic mechanisms. This is because RV-C cannot be propagated using the conventional method that is described for RV-A and RV-B in Chapter 2. H1HeLa cells or primary lung fibroblasts do not express the receptor for RV-C and, therefore, they are resistant to RV-C infection. Recently, human mucociliary-differentiated immortalized airway epithelial cells expressing cadherin-related family member 3 cells were shown to be suitable for propagating RV-C from clinical samples, but this method may not be sustainable due to the costs of culturing the cells for large-scale virus production. Another method to propagate the virus is to transfect the viral genome into H1HeLa or primary lung fibroblasts to bypass the initial infection step, which is the binding and endocytosis of the virus. RV-C virus propagated by this method was demonstrated to yield relatively high-titer infectious virus suitable for in vitro studies. Here, we describe a method to propagate and purify the RV-C suitable for in vitro and in vivo studies.

Key words HeLa cells, Transfection, Ultrafiltration

1 Introduction

Human rhinoviruses (RV) cause respiratory illness ranging from mild, self-limiting upper respiratory infection to severe respiratory disease, particularly in patients with underlying chronic lung diseases such as asthma, chronic obstructive pulmonary disease, and cystic fibrosis [1–4]. RV is the second most common respiratory virus associated with severe bronchiolitis in children [5]. Based on the sequence similarities, RVs were classified into three species: RV-A, RV-B, and RV-C. The pathogenesis and biology of RV-A and RV-B species have been extensively studied both in vitro and in vivo and also through experimental infection in humans [6, 7]. Due to limitations in the propagation of RV-C, not much is known about this virus. However, RV-C has been shown to be

Umadevi Sajjan (ed.), *Rhinovirus: Methods and Protocols*, Methods in Molecular Biology, vol. 2903,
https://doi.org/10.1007/978-1-0716-4410-2_3,

associated with more severe asthma exacerbations in children requiring hospitalization [8–10].

The first step in the propagation of rhinovirus is viral binding to its receptor and gaining entry into the cells. The conventional cell lines, H1HeLa cells, and primary lung fibroblasts (WiSL), used for the propagation of RV-A and RV-B species, do not express the receptor for RV-C, which binds to a human cadherin-related family member (CDHR)3 [11]. The CDHR3 is primarily expressed in ciliated cells of the airway epithelium [12]. Therefore, mucociliary-differentiated nasal epithelial cell cultures and immortalized bronchial epithelial cell lines with the capacity to differentiate have been used to propagate RV-C [13–15]. However, these methods require the culturing of cells for up to 4 weeks in transwells using an expensive medium; therefore, they are not cost-effective. Moreover, the virus yield is low. RV-C was also propagated by transfecting vRNA into either WiSL cells or HeLa cells expressing human CDHR3 C529Y [16, 17]. The virus was purified from the culture supernatant by sucrose cushion ultracentrifugation or ultrafiltration. Here, we describe a cost-effective method to propagate and purify e-high-titer infectious RV-C based on the methods described in [13, 16, 17].

2 Materials

1. HeLa cells (ATCC CRL-1958).
2. Tracheobronchial epithelial cells (Lifeline Technologies Cat # FC-0035).
3. Rhinovirus C15 cDNA [13].
4. Bronchial Life medium (Lifeline Technologies Cat# LL-0023).
5. ROCK inhibitor, Y 27632 (Bio-Techne/Tocris Cat# 1254).
6. Differentiation medium (*see* Ref. 18].
7. Accutase (Innovative Cell Technologies Cat# AT-104).
8. Type I bovine collagen (PureCol, Advanced Biomatrix Cat# 05005).
9. DMEM-high glucose (Gibco, 11,965,092 or equivalent).
10. Fetal bovine serum.
11. Complete medium (DMEM, 1% L-Glutamine, 1% Pen/Strep, 10% Fetal bovine serum).
12. Cell storage medium (Serum-free medium, 10% DMSO, 10% Fetal bovine serum).
13. Trypsin/EDTA: 0.25% (w/v) trypsin/0.02% (w/v) EDTA (Gibco 25,200,056 or equivalent).
14. Sterile cell culture-grade PBS without $CaCl_2$ and $MgCl_2$.

15. Endotoxin-free sterile PBS with $CaCl_2$ and $MgCl_2$ (Gibco).
16. Cell culture incubator set at 37 °C.
17. ZymoPure II Plasmid Maxiprep (Zymo Research).
18. RiboMAX™ Large Scale RNA Production System-T7 (Promega).
19. BstB1 restriction enzyme (New England BioLabs).
20. DNA clean and concentrator kit (ZymoResearch Cat# D4014).
21. RNA clean and concentrator kit (ZymoResearch Cat# R1017).
22. Xfect™ RNA Transfection Reagent (Takara Bio Cat# 631450).
23. 50× 4-(2-hydroxyethyl)-1-piperazineethanesulfonic acid (HEPES) buffer. Dissolve HEPES dry powder to a final concentration of 1.25 M D-PBS and adjust the pH to 7.3–7.4.
24. Lauria-Bertani media (ThermoFisher Scientific).
25. Bacto agar (ThermoFisher Scientific).
26. Molecular biology-grade agarose and TRIS/EDTA acetate buffer (ThermoFisher Scientific).
27. Tris/EDTA/Acetate buffer phAmpicillin (100 mg/mL, ThermoFisher Scientific).
28. 6.5 mm transwells (Corning/Costar Cat# 3460)
29. 100 mm × 15 mm tissue-culture-treated plates
30. 150 mm × 25 mm tissue-culture-treated plates
31. Biosafety Level 2 cell culture hood.
32. A benchtop refrigerated centrifuge.
33. Nanodrop or other UV spectrophotometer.
34. Millipore Amicon Stirred Ultrafiltration Cell (Cat# UFSC40001).
35. 100 kDa cutoff ultrafiltration membranes (Millipore Sigma cat#PLHK07610).
36. Filter units with a 0.45 cutoff membrane.
37. Glass filters to fit the filter units.
38. Sterile 2-mL cryovials.
39. Nitrogen gas tank with regulator.

3 Methods

3.1 Preparation of HeLa Cell Stocks

1. Warm up the complete medium in a 37 °C water bath.
2. Aliquot 10 mL of warm medium into a 15 mL sterile conical tube in a cell culture hood.

3. Thaw a frozen vial of HeLa cells (*see* **Note 1**) in a 37 °C water bath.
4. Sterilize the outside of the vial with 70% ethanol and transfer the vial to cell culture hood.
5. Transfer cells from the vials to a 15 mL centrifuge tube containing 10 mL of warm medium. Invert gently two times to mix the content.
6. Centrifuge for 5 min at 500× *g*, 4 °C, and remove supernatant by aspiration.
7. Resuspend the cell pellet in 1 mL of complete medium and transfer it to a 10-cm cell culture dish containing 10 mL of complete medium. Rotate the dish to evenly distribute the cells.
8. Incubate the cell culture dish in a cell culture incubator at 37 °C. Change the medium every 2 days.
9. When the cells reach 70–80% confluency, aspirate the medium and rinse the plate 2 times with 10 mL PBS without $CaCl_2$ and $MgCl_2$.
10. Add 3 mL of trypsin/EDTA and place it in an incubator for up to 2 min.
11. Tap the plate gently against the palm to release the adherent cells.
12. Add 10 mL of complete medium and transfer cells to a sterile 50-mL centrifuge tube. Add 10 mL PBS to the plate and transfer it to a tube containing the cells.
13. Centrifuge for 5 min at 500× *g*, 4 °C, and remove supernatant by aspiration.
14. Resuspend cell pellet in 5 mL of complete medium by pipetting up and down.
15. Count the cells using a cell counter or hemacytometer and suspend the cells in complete medium to adjust the cell density to 1–3 × 10^6 cells/mL.
16. Plate cells in three 10 cm dishes (5 × 10^5 cells/dish), which will be used in Subheading 3.4.
17. For the cryopreservation of HeLa cells, add DMSO at 10% to the cell suspension. Aliquot 1–2 × 10^6 cells in 1 mL into cryovials and place it in a chilled freezer box at −80 °C.
18. Transfer cryovials into the liquid nitrogen tank for longer-term storage.

3.2 Preparation of Plasmid DNA

1. Prepare 100 μg/mL of ampicillin-containing LB agar plates and LB broth.

2. Culture bacteria containing RV-C15 cDNA on LB agar/ampicillin plates and incubate at 37 °C overnight.
3. Transfer a single colony into 2 mL LB broth containing ampicillin and incubate in a shaker incubator for 8 h at 37 °C—starting culture.
4. Inoculate 100 mL of LB broth/ampicillin with 1 mL of the starter culture and grow overnight in a shaker incubator at 37 °C, 225 rpm.
5. Isolate plasmid using the ZymoPure II plasmid purification kit following the manufacturer's instructions and determine the concentration of plasmid using Nanodrop or UV-spectrophotometer.

3.3 Linearization and Transcription of cDNA

1. Digestion of plasmid with BstB1 restriction enzyme as follows:
   1. 5 μg of cDNA containing plasmid
   2. DNAse-free water (add to make up the volume to 30 μL).
   3. 3 μL of restriction enzyme buffer
   4. 0.9 μL of BstB1 enzyme
   5. Incubate at 37 °C for 5 h.
2. Run the restriction enzyme digest on 0.7% agarose gel in TAE buffer. Visualize the DNA bands with ethidium bromide or similar DNA stain (*see* **Note 2**).
3. Excise the DNA corresponding to linearized plasmid DNA (approximately 10,000 bp) and purify the linearized cDNA by using PCR cleanup and concentrator kit following the manufacturer's instructions and determine the concentration of cDNA by using Nanodrop.
4. Synthesize RNA from the cDNA using Ribomax polymerase as follows.
   1. 2 μg of linearized cDNA
   2. 4 μL Ribomax polymerase buffer
   3. 2 μL 100 mM dithiothreitol
   4. μL RNasin
   5. 1.5 μL Ribomax
   6. RNase/DNase-free water to 20 μL.
   7. Incubate at 37 °C for 3 h.
5. Add 1 μL of RNase-free DNase to the transcription mix and 74 uL of RNase/DNase-free water.
6. Incubate at 37 °C for 20 min.

7. Purify and concentrate the RNA by using an RNA clean up and concentrator kit following the manufacturer's instructions.
8. Determine the concentration of purified RNA by Nanodrop.

3.4 RNA Transfection of HeLa Cells

1. Grow HeLa cells in a 100 cm cell culture dish to 70–80% confluency.
2. On the day of transfection, replace the medium with 6 mL of fresh medium.
3. Prepare the transfection mix as follows for each 100 cm dish.
   1. Tube 1:8 μg of RNA in 50 μL + 500 μL of Xfect reaction buffer mix by vortexing.
   2. Tube 2:50 μL of Xfect RNA transfection polymer +500 μL of Xfect reaction buffer mix well.
   3. Transfer the contents of tube 2 to tube 1. Mix well by vortexing for 5 s at medium speed.
   4. Incubate for 10 min at room temperature to form nanoparticles.
4. Add the entire transfection mix dropwise to the cell culture. Rock the plate gently to mix the contents (*see* **Note 3**).
5. Incubate the plate for 4 h at 37 at 37 °C.
6. Remove the transfection complexes by aspirating the medium. Add 10 mL of fresh medium.
7. Incubate the plate at 37 °C for 48–72 h (*see* **Note 4**) or until the cells show cytopathic effect.
8. Add 200 μL of HEPES buffer to each plate. Freeze the plate at −80 °C. Thaw the plate at room temperature for 30 min until the medium in the plate is completely thawed.
9. Repeat the freeze-thaw cycles two more times.
10. Transfer the cell lysate to a 30 mL sterile centrifuge tube and centrifuge at 6000× *g* for 10 min at 4 °C to remove cell debris.
11. Collect the supernatant into a fresh 50 mL sterile conical tube. Add 100 ul of RNase A/10 mL cell lysate (Stock 10 mg/mL RNase A), and incubate for 10 in at 37 °C to remove transfection input RNA.
12. Subject the supernatant to ultrafiltration using 100,000 kDa cutoff membranes as described in Chapter 2 for RV-A and RV-B. Collect the concentrated virus and store it in aliquots at −80 °C.

3.5 Assessing the Infectivity of the Virus

1. Coat 10 cm dishes with 5 μg of PureCol™/cm^2 in sterile distilled water overnight at 4 °C.
2. Aspirate the liquid and dry the plates under UV light in the cell culture hood for 1 h (*see* **Note 5**).

3. Wash the plates with water two times to remove excess collagen and hydrate the collagen film.
4. Prepare BronchialLife medium by mixing basal medium with BronchialLife Life Factors provided with the kit. Do not add gentamicin and amphotericin that are included in the kit as optional ingredients. Add 5 mL of Penicillin/Streptomycin. Store the medium at 4 °C.
5. Differentiation medium: Please refer to Chapter 9 or Ref. [18]. This medium can also be purchased from Lifeline Technologies (Cat# LM-0050).
6. Aliquot the required volume of BronchialLife medium and warm it in a water bath for 15 min. Add ROCK inhibitor to 5 μM and add 10 mL to a 10 cm collagen-coated dish. ROCK inhibitor should be added fresh to the medium on the day of use.
7. Seed human tracheobronchial epithelial cells (Lifeline Technologies) at a density of 5000 cells/cm^2.
8. Incubate in a cell culture incubator at 37 °C until the cells become 80% to 90% confluent. Change the medium every 2–3 days.
9. Aspirate the medium and wash once with D-PBS.
10. Add 7 mL of cold or room temperature accutase to the plate and incubate at room temperature until the cells detach from the plate.
11. Transfer the cells to a 50 mL sterile conical tube, rinse the plate with 10 mL D-PBS twice, and combine them with the cells.
12. Centrifuge the cell suspension at 500× *g* for 5 min at 4 °C.
13. Aspirate the supernatant and suspend the cell pellet in fresh BronchialLife medium.
14. Determine the density of cells and adjust to 5×10^5 cells/mL with medium.
15. Add 200 μL of cell suspension to the apical chamber of collagen-coated transwells (*see* **Note 6**). Add 0.6 mL of BronchialLife medium to the bottom chamber and grow the cells until they become 100% confluent. Change the medium once in 2–3 days.
16. Remove the medium from the apical chamber and replace the medium in the basolateral chamber with 0.6 mL of differentia tion medium, creating an air/liquid interface (ALI).
17. Maintain the cells at ALI for 4 weeks in the differentiation medium with a changing medium every 2–3 days to promote mucociliary differentiation (*see* **Note 7**) (Fig. 1).

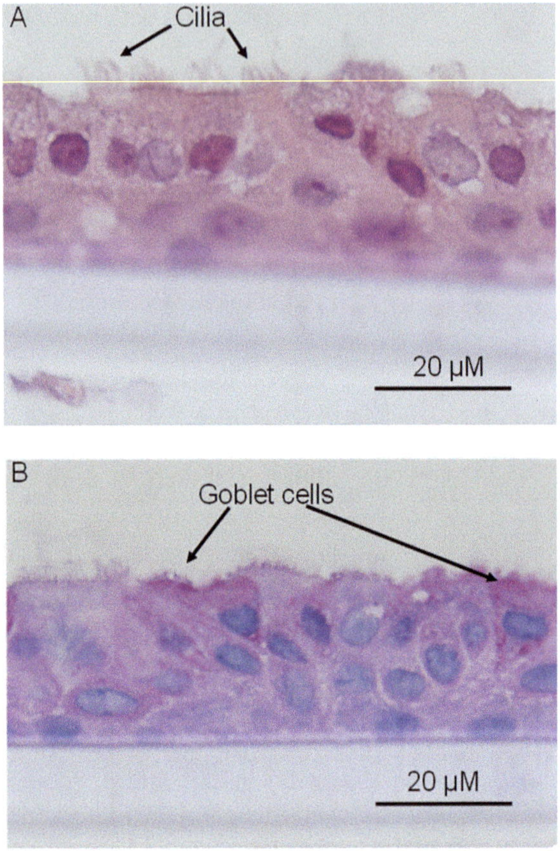

Fig. 1 Cell cultures grown on transwells were embedded in paraffin. Five-micron-thick sections were deparaffinized and stained with either hematoxylin and eosin (**a**) or periodic acid Schiff's reagent to detect goblet cells (**b**)

18. On the day of infection, rinse the apical surface of the cultures with D-PBS to remove the secreted mucus. Transfer the transwells to a new receiver plate containing fresh differentiation medium.
19. Add virus at a multiplicity of infection of 1 (3×10^5 virions) in 10 μL to the apical surface. The control wells should be infected with the same volume of UV-irradiated RV-C15 [19].
20. Incubate for 24 h at 37 °C. Collect the basolateral medium and measure the pro-inflammatory cytokines and type I interferon, IFN-β, and IFN-λ1.
21. Wash the cells with PBS, lyse cells in TRIZOL, extract RNA using a Directzol kit, and determine the viral RNA by qPCR [13, 16].

The propagation method summarized from Refs. [13, 16], combined with ultrafiltration developed by our lab, yields semipurified RV-C, which maintains its infectivity.

This method will yield a partially purified virus which is free of cellular material such as RNA, DNA, cytokines, growth factors, proteases, RNases and DNases, and serum proteins. This partially purified virus is viable, infects airway epithelial cells in vitro and mouse airways in vivo efficiently, and stimulates pro-inflammatory and antiviral effects [19, 20].

4 Notes

1. HeLa cells must be tested for mycoplasma contamination (the mycoplasma detection kit can be purchased from Sigma or other suppliers). Sham generated from mycoplasma-contaminated will stimulate pro-inflammatory responses, which are indistinguishable from RV infection. If the cells are contaminated with mycoplasma, the cells should be cured using the mycoplasma elimination kit (Sigma Aldrich kit Cat#-CUL001B). The cells should be routinely tested for mycoplasma.
2. The circular plasmid DNA will be lower in size compared to linearized DNA.
3. It is not necessary to use serum-free medium. The medium color will change when the transfection mix is added to the cells, and it is normal.
4. At least 50% cytopathic effect is necessary; otherwise, the viral yield will be low.
5. After drying, the collagen-coated plates can be stored at 4 °C, wrapped in cellowrap, for up to 3 months.
6. Coating transwells with PureCol™: Dilute PureCol in distilled water to 1000 μg/mL. Add 50 μL to the apical chamber of the transwell. Incubate overnight at 4 °C. Aspirate the collagen and dry under UV light in a cell culture hood. Wrap the plates in a cellowrap and store at 4 °C.
7. The tracheobronchial epithelial cells cultured at ALI for the first 2–7 days show medium on the apical surface. Once the cells polarize, the apical chamber of the transwells look almost dry, and there will not be any medium. After 3 weeks of culturing, there will be goblet cells, which will secrete mucus, and this will collect in the apical chamber. To remove the mucus, add 0.3 mL PBS every 3–6 days and aspirate the PBS along with the mucus. This should be done carefully to avoid disturbing the cells growing on the transwell membrane. After 4 weeks at ALI, the cultures show abundant beating cilia.

References

1. Makela MJ, Puhakka T, Ruuskanen O, Leinonen M, Saikku P, Kimpimaki M, Blomqvist S, Hyypia T, Arstila P (1998) Viruses and bacteria in the etiology of the common cold. J Clin Microbiol 36:539–542
2. Lee WM, Lemanske RF Jr, Evans MD, Vang F, Pappas T, Gangnon R, Jackson DJ, Gern JE (2012) Human rhinovirus species and season of infection determine illness severity. Am J Respir Crit Care Med 186:886–891
3. Etherington C, Naseer R, Conway SP, Whitaker P, Denton M, Peckham DG (2014) The role of respiratory viruses in adult patients with cystic fibrosis receiving intravenous antibiotics for a pulmonary exacerbation. J Cyst Fibros 13:49–55
4. George SN, Garcha DS, Mackay AJ, Patel AR, Singh R, Sapsford RJ, Donaldson GC, Wedzicha JA (2014) Human rhinovirus infection during naturally occurring COPD exacerbations. Eur Respir J 44:87–96
5. Hasegawa K, Mansbach JM, Camargo CA Jr (2014) Infectious pathogens and bronchiolitis outcomes. Expert Rev Anti-Infect Ther 12: 817–828
6. Jacobs SE, Lamson DM, St George K, Walsh TJ (2013) Human rhinoviruses. Clin Microbiol Rev 26:135–162
7. Mallia P, Message SD, Gielen V, Contoli M, Gray K, Kebadze T, Aniscenko J, Laza-Stanca-V, Edwards MR, Slater L et al (2011) Experimental rhinovirus infection as a human model of chronic obstructive pulmonary disease exacerbation. Am J Respir Crit Care Med 183:734–742
8. Miller EK, Edwards KM, Weinberg GA, Iwane MK, Griffin MR, Hall CB, Zhu Y, Szilagyi PG, Morin LL, Heil LH et al (2009) A novel group of rhinoviruses is associated with asthma hospitalizations. J Allergy Clin Immunol 123(98–104):e101
9. Khetsuriani N, Lu X, Teague WG, Kazerouni N, Anderson LJ, Erdman DD (2008) Novel human rhinoviruses and exacerbation of asthma in children. Emerg Infect Dis 14:1793–1796
10. Bizzintino J, Lee WM, Laing IA, Vang F, Pappas T, Zhang G, Martin AC, Khoo SK, Cox DW, Geelhoed GC et al (2011) Association between human rhinovirus C and severity of acute asthma in children. Eur Respir J 37: 1037–1042
11. Griggs TF, Bochkov YA, Basnet S, Pasic TR, Brockman-Schneider RA, Palmenberg AC, Gern JE (2017) Rhinovirus C targets ciliated airway epithelial cells. Respir Res 18:84
12. Bochkov YA, Watters K, Ashraf S, Griggs TF, Devries MK, Jackson DJ, Palmenberg AC, Gern JE (2015) Cadherin-related family member 3, a childhood asthma susceptibility gene product, mediates rhinovirus C binding and replication. Proc Natl Acad Sci USA 112: 5485–5490
13. Bochkov YA, Palmenberg AC, Lee WM, Rathe JA, Amineva SP, Sun X, Pasic TR, Jarjour NN, Liggett SB, Gern JE (2011) Molecular modeling, organ culture and reverse genetics for a newly identified human rhinovirus C. Nat Med 17:627–632
14. Hao W, Bernard K, Patel N, Ulbrandt N, Feng H, Svabek C, Wilson S, Stracener C, Wang K, Suzich J et al (2012) Infection and propagation of human rhinovirus C in human airway epithelial cells. J Virol 86:13524–13532
15. Nakauchi M, Nagata N, Takayama I, Saito S, Kubo H, Kaida A, Oba K, Odagiri T, Kageyama T (2019) Propagation of rhinovirus C in differentiated immortalized human airway HBEC3-KT epithelial cells. Viruses:11
16. Griggs TF, Bochkov YA, Nakagome K, Palmenberg AC, Gern JE (2015) Production, purification, and capsid stability of rhinovirus C types. J Virol Methods 217:18–23
17. Rajput C, Han M, Ishikawa T, Lei J, Goldsmith AM, Jazaeri S, Stroupe CC, Bentley JK, Hershenson MB (2021) Rhinovirus C infection induces type 2 innate lymphoid cell expansion and eosinophilic airway inflammation. Front Immunol 12:649520
18. Fulcher ML, Gabriel S, Burns KA, Yankaskas JR, Randell SH (2005) Well-differentiated human airway epithelial cell cultures. Methods Mol Med 107:183–206
19. Schneider D, Ganesan S, Comstock AT, Meldrum CA, Mahidhara R, Goldsmith AM, Curtis JL, Martinez FJ, Hershenson MB, Sajjan U (2010) Increased cytokine response of rhinovirus-infected airway epithelial cells in chronic obstructive pulmonary disease. Am J Respir Crit Care Med 182:332–340
20. Newcomb DC, Sajjan U, Nanua S, Jia Y, Goldsmith AM, Bentley JK, Hershenson MB (2005) Phosphatidylinositol 3-kinase is required for rhinovirus-induced airway epithelial cell interleukin-8 expression. J Biol Chem 280: 36952–36961

Chapter 4

Quantification of Infectious Rhinovirus A and B Serotypes by Plaque Assay

Mohsen Tabasi, Haleh Ganjian, and Umadevi Sajjan

Abstract

Plaque assay is a quantitative assay that determines the number of infective virions in the viral stock or the infected cells. Plaques are essentially virus-infected cells that produce progeny virus and infect adjacent cells. The cells producing progeny virus die and detach from the dish, leaving an empty space in the confluent monolayer of cells. Unlike other viruses, rhinovirus does not form characteristic round plaques but shows small clear areas of different shapes surrounded by dying cells. Rhinoviruses form plaques only in highly susceptible H1HeLa cells but not in their primary target, airway epithelial cells. The plaque assay to determine the number of infective virions works only for rhinovirus species A and B, but not C, because the latter does not infect H1HeLa cells. Here we describe a method to quantify the infective virions by plaque assay for rhinovirus speciesA and B.

Key words Virus infectivity assay, H1HeLa cells, Cell death, Crystal violet, Airway epithelial cells, $TCID_{50}$

1 Introduction

Rhinoviruses are small RNA viruses and are responsible for the majority of common colds [1, 2]. Rhinoviruses are also associated with exacerbations in patients with underlying chronic airway diseases, such as asthma, cystic fibrosis, and chronic obstructive pulmonary disease [3–5]. Phylogenetically, approximately 100 different rhinovirus strains have been identified and subdivided into A and B species based on partial sequencing of viral capsid-encoding regions, non-encoding regions, and a limited number of complete genomes [6]. Highly sensitive molecular techniques developed for RV detection led to identification of third species and designated as RV-C [7]. Most of RV-A and RV-B strains (major group RV) enter the human airway epithelial cells via human ICAM-1, indicating the species specificity [8]. A minority of RV-A and RV-B strains (major group virus) enter both human

Umadevi Sajjan (ed.), *Rhinovirus: Methods and Protocols*, Methods in Molecular Biology, vol. 2903,
https://doi.org/10.1007/978-1-0716-4410-2_4,

and mouse airway epithelial cells by binding to low-density lipoprotein (LDL) receptors and LDLR-like receptors [9]. RV-C binds to cadherin-related family member 3, which is expressed primarily in ciliated cells [10]. However, unlike respiratory syncytial virus, RV infection seldom causes cytopathic effects in airway epithelial cells.

RV-A and RV-B species, but not RV-C, infect human primary fibroblasts, MRC-5 and WI-38, as well as a clone of the HeLa cell line known as H1HeLa cells. All these three cell types are routinely used to propagate RV [11]. After infection, RV-A and RV-B species cause cytopathic effects in all three cell types, which are visible under the microscope. MRC-5 and WI-38 maintain healthy morphology and show no cell death for up to 4 weeks in culture; therefore, these cells are used in clinical microbiology laboratories for endpoint dilution assays of clinical strains related to RV-A and RV-B. This is because clinical isolates of RV may take longer than a week to induce observable plaques. However, these cells are less than optimal for determining the infectivity of RV in a research laboratory because they do not stain well with crystal violet to quantify the cytopathic effect. On the other hand, H1HeLa cells are highly sensitive to RV-A and RV-B infection and show cytopathic effects within 24–48 h of infection. These cells also stain well with crystal violet. However, although the viral load can be determined by quantifying the viral RNA, there are no appropriate cells to propagate and determine the infectivity of RV-C.

Routinely, the 50% tissue culture infectivity dose ($TCID_{50}$), as determined by cytopathic assay, is used for quantifying the infectivity dose of RV-A and RV-B because these species do not form the characteristic plaques that are observed with other plaque-forming viruses. Since RV-A and RV-B species cause cytopathic effects, a plaque assay was developed using H1HeLa cell and is described here to more accurately titer the viral stock.

2 Materials

1. H1HeLa cells (ATCC CRL-1958).
2. Humidified, 37 °C, 5% CO_2 incubator.
3. Humidified, 33 °C, 5% CO_2 incubator.
4. −80 °C freezer
5. Water bath.
6. Microwave.
7. Liquid nitrogen tank.
8. Sterile disposables for tissue culture.
9. 100-mm dishes
10. 6-well plates

11. 50-mL sterile capped tubes
12. 1.5-mL sterile microfuge tubes
13. 10-mL sterile pipettes
14. 5-mL sterile pipettes
15. 2-mL sterile aspirating pipettes
16. 1 mL sterile pipette tips
17. 0.2 mL sterile pipette tips
18. 20 uL sterile pipette tips
19. 2-mL cryovials
20. DMEM-high glucose (Gibco, 11965092 or equivalent).
21. Fetal bovine serum (Cytiva, SH30080.03).
22. Penicillin/Streptomycin (10,000 U/mL) (Gibco, 15140148).
23. L-glutamine (200 mM) (Gibco, A2916801).
24. 1 M Magnesium chloride ($MgCl_2$)—filter sterilized
25. PBS without calcium and magnesium.
26. HBSS with calcium and magnesium.
27. Trypsin-EDTA (0.25%) (Gibco, 25200056).
28. Cell culture grade factor V bovine serum albumin (Sigma, A7638).

    To make up 10% BSA—Dissolve 10 g of BSA in PBS without calcium and magnesium and filter sterilize.
29. Ultrapure low melting point (LMP) agarose (ThermoFisher Scientific, 16520050).
30. Complete medium: 500 mL DMEM medium +5 mL of L-glutamine +5 mL of Pen/strep +50 mL of FBS.
31. Supplemental medium: 47.5 mL complete medium +2 mL 1 M $MgCl_2$ + 0.5 mL 10% BSA.
32. Top agarose stock: Suspend 2.5 g of ultrapure LMP Agarose in 50 mL of HBSS in a 250 mL bottle, autoclave, and aliquot 6 mL into 50 mL sterile tubes and store at 4 °C. Each 6 mL is sufficient for four 6-well plates. If using less than 6 well plates or 24 well format assays, store the top agarose in smaller aliquots as necessary.
33. Overlay agarose: Preheat supplemental medium at 45 °C. Melt 6 mL agarose stock in a 50 mL tube by briefly heating it in a microwave. Add 44 mL of supplemental preheated medium and place in a water bath set at 45 °C to maintain the temperature until needed. Prepare the overlay agarose just before infecting the cells with the virus. This overlay agarose should be prepared on the day of use. Repeated heating and warming up will destroy the cross-linking ability of the agarose in the

presence of serum and other salts in the medium and will not solidify.

34. Virus dilution buffer: 50 mL HBSS with magnesium and calcium +1 mL 10% BSA.
35. 3.4% Formaldehyde in PBS—Dilute 37% formaldehyde to 3.4% in PBS
36. Crystal violet solution for staining plaques (0.1% crystal violet in 20% ethanol): Prepare a 10× stock solution by dissolving 1 g of crystal violet in 100 mL of ethanol. Dilute 10–100 mL in distilled water before use. Stock crystal violet solution forms crystals over time. It can be filtered through a glass fiber filter prior to dilution.

3 Methods

3.1 Culturing H1HeLa Cells

1. Warm complete medium in a 37 °C water bath.
2. Aliquot 10 mL of warm medium into a 15 mL sterile conical tube in a cell culture hood.
3. Thaw a frozen vial of HeLa cells in a 37 °C water bath.
4. Sterilize the outside of the vial with 70% ethanol and transfer the vial to the cell culture hood.
5. Transfer cells from the vials to a 15 mL centrifuge tube containing 10 mL of warm medium. Invert gently two times to mix the content.
6. Centrifuge for 5 min at 500× *g*, 4 °C, and remove supernatant by aspiration.
7. Resuspend the pellet in 1 mL of complete medium and transfer it to a 10-cm cell culture dish containing 10 mL of complete medium. Rotate the dish to evenly distribute the cells.
8. Incubate the cell culture dish in a humidified, 5% CO_2 incubator at 37 °C. Change the medium every 2 days until the cells become 70–80% confluent.
9. When the cells reach 70–80% confluency, aspirate the medium and rinse the plate 2 times with 10 mL PBS without $CaCl_2$ and $MgCl_2$ each time.
10. Add 3 mL of trypsin/EDTA and place it in an incubator for up to 2 min.
11. Tap the plate gently against the palm to release the adherent cells.
12. Add 10 mL of complete medium and transfer cells to a sterile 50-mL centrifuge tube. Add 10 mL PBS to the plate and transfer it to a tube containing the cells.

13. Centrifuge for 5 min at 500× *g*, 4 °C, and remove supernatant by aspiration.
14. Resuspend the cell pellet in 5 mL of complete medium by pipetting up and down.
15. Determine the cell number in the cell suspension by using a hemocytometer and adjust the cell density to 1×10^6 cells/4 mL in complete medium.

3.2 Plaque Assay Day 1 Seeding Cells in 6-Well Plates

1. Seed 0.5×10^6 cells in 2 mL per well of complete medium. Calculate the number of wells depending upon the dilution series to be tested in triplicates.
2. Incubate for 24–48 h. The cells should be an even monolayer of 85–90% confluency. Completely (100%) confluent monolayers will not allow enough time for the plaques to fully develop.

3.3 Day 2 to 3 Infection of 85–90% Confluent Monolayer with Virus

1. Prepare a 1:10 serial dilution series of the virus in virus dilution buffer as shown in Fig. 1.
2. Aspirate growth medium from 6-well plates.
3. Add 500 uL of diluted virus per well in triplicates. Gently rock the plate to evenly distribute the inoculum on the cell surface.
4. Incubate for 1 h at 33 °C. Rock the plates gently at 15-min interval.
5. In the meantime, prepare the overlay agarose and maintain it at 45 °C.
6. Tilt the plate to a 45-degree angle and aspirate the inoculum from the edge of the well, taking care not to touch the cell monolayer.
7. Immediately add 2 mL of overlay agarose gently to each well using a 25 mL serological pipette. While adding the overlay

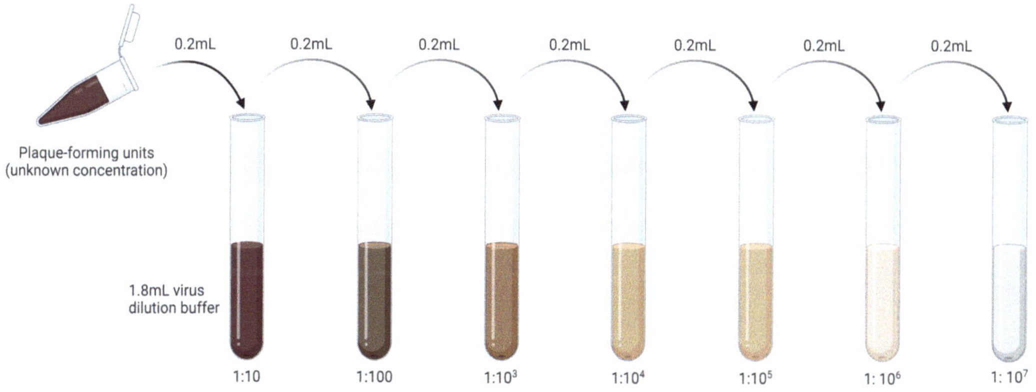

Fig. 1 Preparing 1:10 dilution series of virus stock

agarose, tilt the plate to 45° angle and add the agarose at the lower edge of the wells, then level the plate to let it flow over the surface (1 tube of 50 mL of agarose is sufficient for 4 six-well plates).

8. Leave the plates for 10–15 min at room temperature to allow the agarose to set and transfer the plates to a 33 °C cell culture incubator.

3.4 Day 4 to 6 Plaque Formation and Staining with Crystal Violet

1. Monitor the cells under a light microscope at low magnification. The infected cells show cytopathic areas within 24–48 h and appear as small spherical cells around the plaques (Fig. 2a). Incubate until the cytopathic areas are clearly visible (Fig. 2b).
2. Add 2 mL of PBS on the surface of the agarose and carefully remove the agarose with a 10 mL serological pipette, taking care not to disturb the cell monolayer.
3. Add 2 mL of 3.4% formaldehyde and incubate for 30 min at room temperature to fix the cells.
4. Flick the plate to remove the formaldehyde and add 2 mL of 0.1% crystal violet and incubate for 10 min at room temperature.
5. Carefully aspirate the stain from the side of the well and then keep the plate inverted on a paper towel to remove the remaining stain.
6. Count the number of colonies at each dilution. The plaques should be visible as clear areas (Fig. 3).
7. The infectious viral titer is calculated as below.

   PFU/mL = Average number of plaques from triplicate wells × 2 (volume of infectious virus added per well) × Dilution factor.

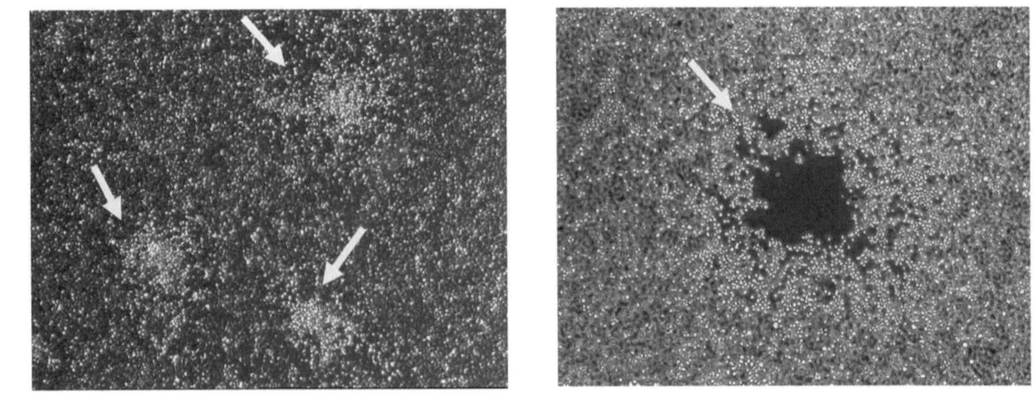

Fig. 2 Plaques formed by RV-A16. (**a**) White highlighted areas (arrow) showing the cytopathic areas with spherical cells at 24 post-infection (**b**) arrow shows a clear plaque surrounded by small spherical dead cells at 72 h post-infection

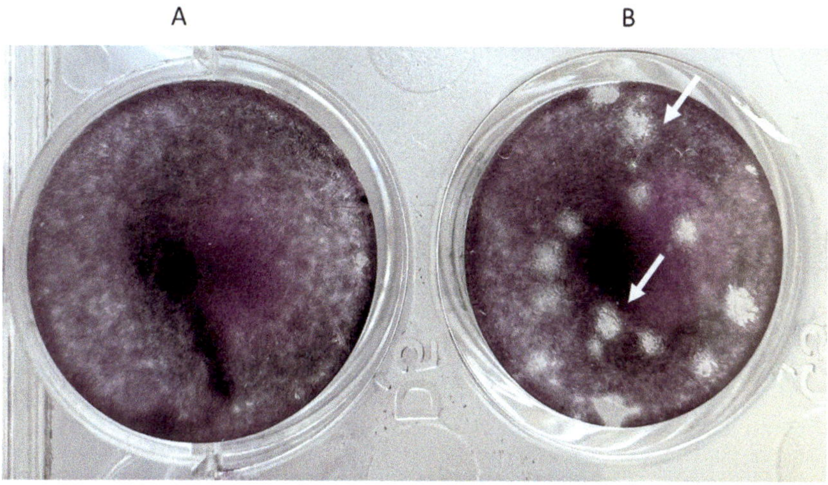

Fig. 3 Crystal violet-stained H1-HeLa cells showing plaques formed by RV-A16. (**a**) Control uninfected cells and (**b**) cells infected with RV-A16 showing plaques (white unstained area, arrow)

4 Notes

1. The purified virus often forms clumps. Make sure to disperse the virus by gently vortexing and pipetting up and down several times. If using cells, subject cells along with spent medium to 2 rounds of freeze-thaw to release the intracellular virus. Centrifuge the cell lysate at 500× *g* to remove the cell debris. Use the supernatant to determine viral titer.
2. Prepare a 1:10 serial dilution series of the virus in sterile HBSS (+Ca, +Mg) with 0.2% FBS. When preparing serial dilutions of the virus, change the pipette tips to avoid carryover of the virus and vortex the tube thoroughly to mix the viral particles.
3. For triplicate assays, the dilution series can be made at the same time using a 96-well plate.
4. Passage H1HeLa cells at least once prior to seeding the cells in 6-well plates for plaque assay to get an even monolayer of cells. Do not use the cells if there are big senescent cells, which may fall off during plaque assay and may look like a plaque after crystal violet staining. The senescent cells can be differentiated from the real plaque under the microscope prior to staining with crystal violet because the senescent cells are not surrounded by dying cells.
5. While aspirating the medium or agarose from the plate, avoid touching the cell monolayer because the touched area can appear as plaque.

6. The assay can be modified to fit a 24-well plate:
   1. Seed H1HeLa cells at 1×10^5 cells/well.
   2. Infect with 0.3 mL of virus.
   3. Overlay with 0.5 mL agarose.
   4. Fix with 0.5 formaldehyde.
   5. Stain with 0.5 mL crystal violet.

References

1. van der Zalm MM, Wilbrink B, van Ewijk BE, Overduin P, Wolfs TF, van der Ent CK (2011) Highly frequent infections with human rhinovirus in healthy young children: a longitudinal cohort study. J Clin Virol 52:317–320
2. Arruda E, Pitkaranta A, Witek TJ Jr, Doyle CA, Hayden FG (1997) Frequency and natural history of rhinovirus infections in adults during autumn. J Clin Microbiol 35:2864–2868
3. Jackson DJ, Gern JE (2022) Rhinovirus infections and their roles in asthma: etiology and exacerbations. J Allergy Clin Immunol Pract 10:673–681
4. George SN, Garcha DS, Mackay AJ, Patel AR, Singh R, Sapsford RJ, Donaldson GC, Wedzicha JA (2014) Human rhinovirus infection during naturally occurring COPD exacerbations. Eur Respir J 44:87–96
5. de Almeida MB, Zerbinati RM, Tateno AF, Oliveira CM, Romao RM, Rodrigues JC, Pannuti CS, da Silva Filho LV (2010) Rhinovirus C and respiratory exacerbations in children with cystic fibrosis. Emerg Infect Dis 16:996–999
6. Palmenberg AC, Spiro D, Kuzmickas R, Wang S, Djikeng A, Rathe JA, Fraser-Liggett CM, Liggett SB (2009) Sequencing and analyses of all known human rhinovirus genomes reveal structure and evolution. Science 324: 55–59
7. Lamson D, Renwick N, Kapoor V, Liu Z, Palacios G, Ju J, Dean A, St George K, Briese T, Lipkin WI (2006) MassTag polymerase-chain-reaction detection of respiratory pathogens, including a new rhinovirus genotype, that caused influenza-like illness in New York state during 2004-2005. J Infect Dis 194:1398–1402
8. Greve JM, Davis G, Meyer AM, Forte CP, Yost SC, Marlor CW, Kamarck ME, McClelland A (1989) The major human rhinovirus receptor is ICAM-1. Cell 56:839–847
9. Hofer F, Gruenberger M, Kowalski H, Machat H, Huettinger M, Kuechler E, Blaas D (1994) Members of the low density lipoprotein receptor family mediate cell entry of a minor-group common cold virus. Proc Natl Acad Sci USA 91:1839–1842
10. Bochkov YA, Watters K, Ashraf S, Griggs TF, Devries MK, Jackson DJ, Palmenberg AC, Gern JE (2015) Cadherin-related family member 3, a childhood asthma susceptibility gene product, mediates rhinovirus C binding and replication. Proc Natl Acad Sci USA 112: 5485–5490
11. Fenters JD, Fordyce PA, Gerin JL, Holper JC (1967) Propagation of rhinovirus on WI-38 cell monolayers in rolling bottles. Appl Microbiol 15:1460–1464

Chapter 5

Quantifying Rhinovirus Genomic and Negative-Strand RNA by RT-PCR

Shahina Wiehler, Michelle E. Love, and David Proud

Abstract

Molecular methods permit measurements of viral genomic RNA as well as of the negative-strand template generated during rhinovirus replication. As such, assays of negative-strand RNA can provide a means for relative quantification of levels of double-stranded RNA that is generated during replication and that interacts with pattern recognition receptors to activate the host immune response. Here we provide RT-PCR protocols for quantitative assays for rhinovirus genomic and negative-strand RNAs.

Key words Human rhinovirus, Airway epithelium, Real-time PCR genomic RNA, Negative-strand RNA

1 Introduction

Infections with rhinoviruses are responsible for most common colds experienced each year. Moreover, rhinovirus (RV) infections can cause acute exacerbations in patients with lower airway diseases [1]. Measurement of RV replication is necessary to monitor viral pathogenesis and to monitor virus levels in biological fluids and infected cells. Although viral titers remain the "gold standard" for quantifying infectious rhinovirus virions released into airway secretions or epithelial supernatants, these assays are time—consuming, taking up to 6 days to complete, and different cell types need to be used for different viral strains. In addition, this approach cannot currently be used to quantify RV-C strains, as these strains do not infect or cause lysis in any of the standard cell culture lines used for viral titer assays [2]. Given these limitations, molecular methods have become more popular to monitor levels of viral RNA. Although the criticism can be made that levels of RNA may not equate with the final number of infectious virions, these assays permit more detailed temporal analyses of intracellular viral loads as well as of levels of viral RNA in biological fluids. In general, these

Umadevi Sajjan (ed.), *Rhinovirus: Methods and Protocols*, Methods in Molecular Biology, vol. 2903,
https://doi.org/10.1007/978-1-0716-4410-2_5,

assays are more sensitive than traditional viral titer assays, and, in our experience, data obtained correlate well with titer values. RT-PCR approaches were initially developed to quantify levels of the positive-sense genomic strand of rhinoviruses. Assays can be developed either with the goal of detecting multiple/all strains of RV or to detect a single strain of RV, although some challenges exist for both. During RV replication, however, negative strands of RNA are generated and serve as templates for the replication of multiple genomic strands of RNA [3]. In the process, double-stranded RNA (dsRNA) is generated and is recognized by pattern recognition receptors, leading to the activation of proinflammatory and antiviral responses [4]. Although the presence of dsRNA can be detected in cells using immunofluorescent approaches with antibodies to dsRNA [5, 6], such assays are not quantitative. Recently, however, RT-PCR methods have been developed to quantify RV negative-strand levels [7], thereby providing a method of relative quantification of viral dsRNA load in cells. Here, we describe protocols for quantifying levels of RV genomic and negative-strand RNAs.

2 Materials

1. Growth media: Airway Epithelial Cell Basal Medium plus additives provided in the growth medium kit creates a serum-free complete epithelial growth medium (PromoCell). To the medium, add gentamicin (50 μg/mL: Invitrogen), penicillin (100 U/mL), streptomycin (100 μg/mL), and amphotericin B (0.25 μg/mL: Invitrogen).
2. Pre-incubation media: Made in exactly the same way as the growth medium except omitting the hydrocortisone supplement.

3 Methods

The following steps are involved in quantifying rhinovirus RNA (Fig. 1):

1. Sample generation.
2. Sample collection.
3. Isolate RNA.
4. Generate cDNA.
5. Real time PCR.
6. Analyze data.

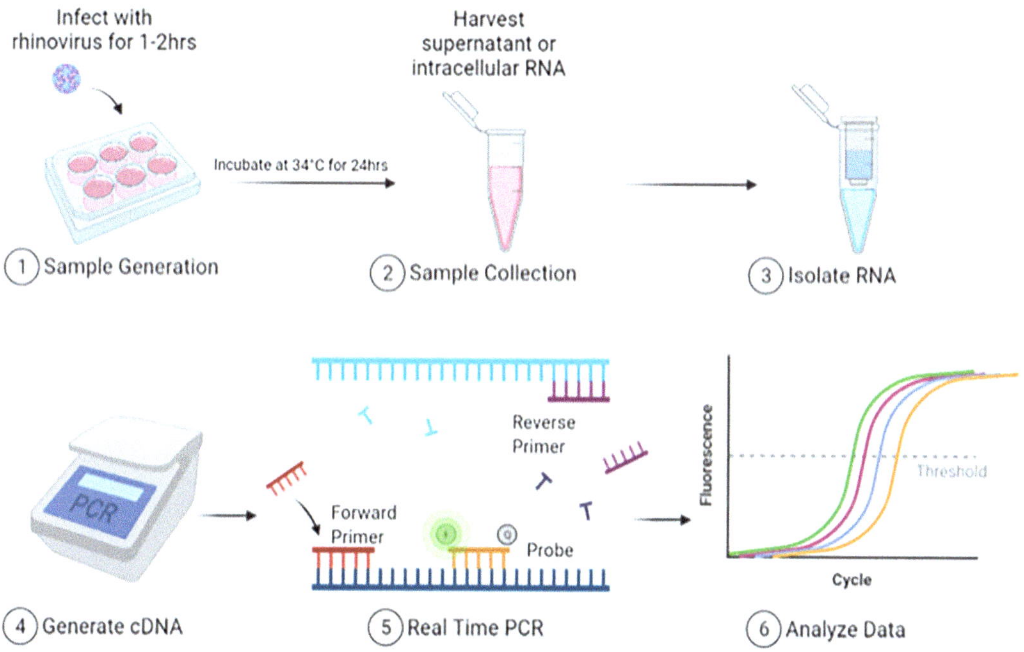

Fig. 1 Workflow for quantifying rhinovirus RNA

3.1 Sample Generation and Collection

The sample preparation described here is for submersion culture of epithelial cell lines or primary human bronchial epithelial cells (HBE) infected with RV-16 and grown in a 6-well plate. Similar procedures can be adapted for other cell systems, such as Air-Liquid Interface (ALI) cultures. All tubes and reagents should be RNase/DNase-free, and proper molecular biology techniques should be followed.

1. Grow submersion epithelial cells in growth medium (1 mL/well), replacing the medium every other day until ~60% confluent.
2. Add 1 mL/well of pre-incubation medium 24 h prior to viral exposure.
3. Add a desired $TCID_{50}$ of RV-16 for 1–2 h. Incubate plates at 34 °C (5% CO_2; 95% humidity) (*see* **Note 1**).
4. Wash cell monolayers three times with 1 mL of HBSS per well to remove any excess input virus.
5. Add 1 mL of fresh pre-incubation media to each well and incubate cells at 34 °C (5% CO_2; 95% humidity) for 24 h (*see* **Note 2**).
6. To quantify virus released into the media, harvest, aliquot, and freeze supernatants at −80 °C.

7. To quantify intracellular virus, wash monolayers with HBSS to remove non-adherent cells and lyse cells immediately in RNA lysis buffer containing chaotropic ions and store lysates at −80 °C (*see* **Note 3**).

3.2 RNA Isolation and cDNA Generation

1. Isolate viral RNA from RV-16 infected supernatant sample or from a preparation of RV-16 using the QIAamp Viral RNA Mini Kit (Qiagen). Follow the manufacturer's protocol, except elute RNA using 60 μL of dH_2O and not with 60 μL of AVE buffer.
2. To isolate intracellular viral RNA, use the NucleoSpin RNA kit (Macherey-Nagel) and elute RNA with 40 μL dH_2O. Quantify RNA using a NanoDrop 2000 (Thermo Fisher Scientific).
3. Reverse transcribe the maximum volume of RNA obtained from a supernatant sample or from a virus preparation with a standard cDNA kit. Follow the manufacturer's protocol (*see* **Note 4**).
4. Reverse transcribe 1 μg of total intracellular RNA with a standard cDNA kit according to the manufacturer's protocol.

3.3 Rhinovirus Real-Time PCR

1. **To Detect Multiple Strains:**

   For several purposes, such as screening samples from a study of naturally acquired colds, an assay that detects multiple/all known strains of RV is particularly helpful. Such an assay is also required for any purpose where the strain of RV present is unknown. To detect multiple RV strains, we designed a quantitative real-time RT-PCR assay targeted to the highly conserved 5′ untranslated region of the RV genome [8], and we have shown that this assay detects several strains from all three RV species: RV-A, RV-B, and RV-C. The strains we used to validate the assay also utilize different receptors for viral entry into cells. It should be noted that the only way to absolutely guarantee that such a system recognizes all strains of RV would be to run every known RV strain (plus new ones as they are isolated) in the assay. Since this would require obtaining an isolate of all known strains and then running each, this would be extremely difficult and time-consuming. As an alternative approach, we performed BLAST searches to determine if one or both of our forward and reverse primers align with all sequences known and, as mentioned, screened several strains from each species, focusing on strains that show sequence variations within each species. After aligning the 5′ untranslated region of all available RV sequences, we designed two forward and two reverse primers to cover minor sequence variations among strains and combined these with a single labeled TaqMan probe (Table 1).

Table 1
Primer and probe sequences to detect multiple RV serotypes

Primer/probe	Sequence
Forward primer 1	5′-AGCCTGCGTGGCTGCC-3′
Forward primer 2	5′-AGCCTGCGTGGCGGC-3′
Reverse primer 1	5′-ACACCCAAAGTAGTCGGTCCC-3′
Reverse primer 2	5′-ACACCCAAAGTAGTTGGTCCCA-3′
Probe (FAM/MGB)	5′-TCCGGCCCCTGAAT-3′

Table 2
Rhinovirus Master Mix

Master mix component	Volume for 1 reaction (μL)
FastStart universal probe master mix	5
dH_2O	0.7
Forward primer 1 (10 μM)	0.4
Forward primer 2 (10 μM)	0.4
Reverse primer 1 (10 μM)	0.4
Reverse primer 2 (10 μM)	0.4
Probe (FAM/MGB) (10 μM)	0.2

First, synthesize all primers and the probe listed in Table 1, and dilute them to a stock concentration of 10 μM in RNase/DNase-free water and aliquot. Store the aliquots at either −20 °C or − 80 °C. Quantification will depend on a synthetic oligonucleotide of known concentration that essentially contains the sequence of the amplicon that will be generated during the RT-PCR reaction. See Subheading 3.4 below.

2. **To Perform the Assay:**
   1. Thaw primers, probe, cDNA samples, and FastStart Universal Probe Master Mix (Rox) (Sigma) and keep them on ice.
   2. All samples will be run in triplicate. Make enough PCR Master Mix to accommodate all samples, plus one more reaction for pipetting error (Table 2). Mix well, briefly (10–15 s) centrifuge droplets to the bottom of the tube in a microfuge and place on ice.
   3. For each individual sample well, take 0.4 μL of cDNA and dilute up to 2.5 μL using dH_2O. Each sample will be run in triplicate, so we suggest using 1.6 μL of cDNA up to 10 μL to give some left after pipetting. Mix well, briefly centrifuge droplets down, and place on ice.

4. Add 7.5 μL Rhinovirus Master Mix into each well of a MicroAmp™ Fast Optical 96-well Reaction Plate (Invitrogen).
5. Add 2.5 μL diluted cDNA to the Rhinovirus Master Mix and mix by pipetting up and down.
6. Load remaining samples.
7. Seal the top of the plate with a MicroAmp™ Optical Adhesive Film (Invitrogen) and briefly spin the plate at 400× *g*. Ensure there are no air bubbles trapped at the bottom of the well. If so, spin the plate again until they are gone.
8. Run the plate on an Applied Biosystems 7500 Fast Real-Time PCR machine (ThermoFisher) under the following PCR cycling conditions: 50 °C for 2 mins, 95 °C for 10 mins, then 40 cycles: 95 °C for 15 s, and 60 °C for 1 min.
9. When the run is complete, average the triplicate cycle threshold (Ct) values for each sample.

3. **To Detect a Single Strain:**

For certain purposes it is desirable to have an assay that detects a single strain of RV. For example, if it is known that experimental infection studies (in vitro or in vivo) will be conducted using a single strain and confirmation of infection with that strain is desired. To detect a specific RV strain, it is advisable to develop primers and probe targeting the highly variable VP1 region of the RV genome, trying to detect a unique sequence for the strain in question. Again, the only way to absolutely ensure that no other strains are detected (if this is likely to be an issue) is to screen all known RV strains in the assay. Given the difficulty and time this would entail, an alternative approach is to perform BLAST searches with the primers and focus on testing strains that have homology to both the forward and reverse primers. Once primers and probe are identified, the remainder of the process is identical to that described above for the multiple strain assay.

3.4 Quantifying Rhinovirus RNA

1. To correlate Ct values to $TCID_{50}$ equivalents, take a purified rhinovirus strain that is known to be detected in the assay used (for the multiple rhinovirus assay we use RV-16). Using a preparation of known titer, isolate the RNA, make cDNA, and dilute the cDNA in half logs to generate a 5-point standard curve.
2. Run a rhinovirus real-time PCR reaction and correlate Ct values to $TCID_{50}$.
3. To quantify the amount of RV to an absolute value, have synthesized a synthetic oligonucleotide sequence containing

the rhinovirus amplicon with two base pairs added to both the 5′ and 3′ ends. The concentration of the synthetic amplicon should be known. For RV-16, this amplicon sequence is:

4. 5′ CTAGCCTGCGTGGCTGCCTGCACACCCACTGGGT GTGAAGCCAAGTATTGGACAAGGTGTGAAGAGCCGC GTGTGCTCATCTTGAGTCCTCCGGCCCCTGAATGTG GCTAACCTTAAACCTGCAGCCAGTGCACACAATCCA GTGTGTAGCTGGTCGTAATGAGCAATTGCGGGATGG GACCAACTACTTTGGGTGTCC-3′.

   Dilute the standard to a concentration of 1000 fg in a volume of 2.5 μL. This should be added to 7.5 μL of master mix in the assay plate. Run standards in triplicate. Using 100-fold dilutions, generate a 6-point standard curve. We recommend running this several times and averaging the data to generate a master standard curve.

5. Use the standard as the template and run an RV real-time PCR reaction. Correlate Ct values to absolute fg amounts (Fig. 2).

   Convert average Ct values to fg using the equation of the line in Fig. 2:

   $y = -1.625\ln(x) + 30.75$, solve for x.

   $y = \text{Ct}$.

   $x = $ sample fg value.

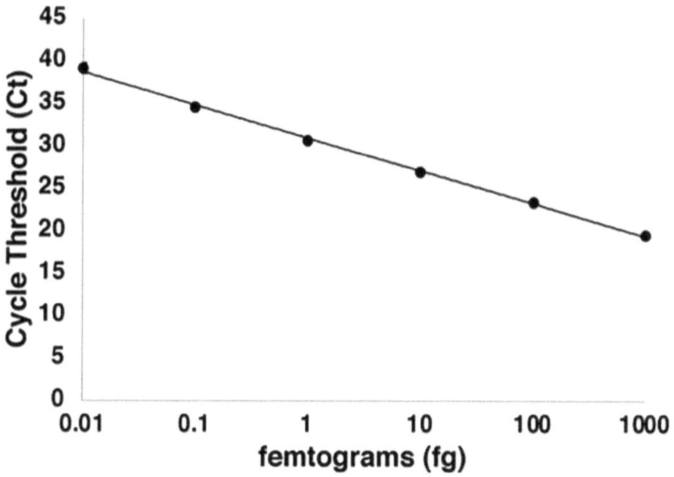

Fig. 2 RV-16 real-time PCR standard curve. Serial dilutions of a synthetic rhinovirus amplicon were used as a template and run in the rhinovirus real-time PCR assay. The equation of the line is: $y = -1.625\ln(x) + 30.75$. Data are mean ± SEM ($n = 3$)

These absolute amounts can also be converted to copy number as follows:

Copy number calculation*:

Copy number = (Sample fg value $\times$ 6.022 $\times$ 10^{23})/(195 bp $\times$ 660 g/mol $\times$ 1 $\times$ 10^{15}).

Avogadro's number = 6.022 $\times$ 10^{23}.

Amplicon size = 195 bp.

Molecular weight of DNA = 660 g/mol.

*This is a base calculation. If determining the copy number from the initial sample is desired then you would multiply the copy number by the RNA concentration for that sample as well as factor in all the dilutions you made during the RNA isolation, cDNA generation and real-time PCR steps.

3.5 Negative-Strand Sample Preparation

1. It has been clearly shown for each of several single-strand positive sense viruses that conventional RT-PCR using primers to the virus strand cannot be used to reliably quantify negative-strand RNA [9, 10], particularly when excess positive strand genomic RNA is present [11]. This is because of the phenomenon of "self-priming" in which signal is generated by positive strand even when primer is omitted from the reverse transcription reaction. To overcome this effect the assay utilizes a chimeric primer during the reverse transcription reaction. This chimeric primer contains a non-viral sequence at the 5′-end of the specific sequence targeting the negative strand of rhinovirus. This non-viral sequence is used as a primer to amplify the negative strand during the PCR step.
2. To determine the amount of negative-strand RV-16 template that is within a cell, briefly expose epithelial cells to RV-16, isolate intracellular RNA and quantify RNA as described above in Subheadings 3.1 and 3.2.

Table 3
Primer and probe sequences used for the negative-strand RV-16 Real-Time PCR reaction

Name	Purpose of oligonucleotide	Sequence
Neg-tag-cDNA primer	Chimeric RT primer	5′-<u>ATCAGCGATGCCGAACGTAT</u> GGCAGCATGGG CAACCT-3′
For RV-16 primer	Real-time PCR forward primer	5′-TGCTGATGCAATACTCAAAAAGG-3′
Tag-rev primer	Real-time PCR reverse primer	5'-<u>ATCAGCGATGCCGAACGTAT</u>-3'
Negative probe	Real-time PCR probe	5′FAM-TGAAAAGCGAGGGA-MGB3′

Underlined nucleotides denotes the non-viral tag sequence

Table 4
Negative-strand master mix

Master mix component	Volume for 1 reaction (μL)
FastStart universal probe master mix	5
For RV-16 primer (10 μM)	1
Tag-rev primer (10 μM)	1
Negative probe (FAM/MGB) (10 μM)	0.5

3. Reverse transcribe RNA using Maxima Reverse Transcriptase (Invitrogen) (*see* **Note 5**). For each reaction mix on ice 1 μg RNA, 1 μL 20 pmol Neg-Tag-cDNA primer (*see* **Note 6**) (Table 3), 1 μL 10 mM dNTP and add enough dH_2O to bring the total reaction volume to 14.5 μL. Mix well.
4. In a thermocycler, incubate the reaction at 65 °C for 1 minute then 4 °C for an additional minute. Briefly centrifuge and place tubes on ice.
5. Make a master mix containing 4 μL 5× RT Buffer, 0.5 μL dH_2O, and 1 μL Maxima Reverse Transcriptase. Add 5.5 μL of this master mix to each reaction.
6. Incubate at 65 °C for 30 mins (*see* **Note 7**), 85 ° C for 5 mins and then hold at 4 °C.
7. To remove any excess RNA template, add 1 μL RNase Cocktail™ Enzyme Mix (Invitrogen) and mix.
8. Incubate at 37 °C for 30 mins.
9. To remove any excess reverse transcription primer, purify cDNA with the QIAquick® PCR Purification Kit (Qiagen). Follow manufacturer's protocol except elute DNA with 30 μL dH_2O.

3.6 Negative-Strand Real-Time PCR

1. Make negative-strand master mix (Table 4).
2. Dilute cDNA 1:2 in dH_2O. Each reaction requires 2.5 μL diluted cDNA. Make enough diluted cDNA to run each sample in triplicate plus one extra reaction. Mix well, briefly centrifuge any droplets down and place on ice.
3. Add 7.5 μL Negative-Strand Master Mix into each well of a MicroAmp™ Fast Optical 96-well Reaction Plate.
4. Add 2.5 μL diluted cDNA to the Negative-Strand Master Mix and mix by pipetting up and down.
5. Load remaining samples.
6. Seal the top of the plate with a MicroAmp™ Optical Adhesive Film and briefly spin the plate at 400× *g*. Ensure there are no

air bubbles trapped at the bottom of the well. If so, spin the plate again until they are gone.

7. Run the plate on an Applied Biosystems 7500 Fast Real-Time PCR machine under the following PCR cycling conditions: 50 °C for 2 mins, 95 °C for 10 mins, then 40 cycles: 95 °C for 15 s and 60 °C for 1 min.
8. Average the triplicate cycle threshold (Ct) values for each sample.

3.7 Quantifying Negative-Strand RNA

1. To quantify the amount of negative strand to an absolute value, synthesize a synthetic negative-strand oligonucleotide that includes the amplicon sequence with five base pairs added to both the 5′ and 3′ ends. The concentration of this standard will be known. For Rhinovirus change Rhinovirus to RV-16 the negative-strand amplicon is: 5′TAATAATCAGCGATGCC GAACGTATGGCAGCATGGGCAACCTTTCCCTCGCTTTT CACTTCCCTTTTTGAGTATTGCATCAGCAAAAAT3′.
2. Dilute the standard to a concentration of 100 fg in a volume of 2.5 μL. This should be added to 7.5 μL of master mix in the assay plate. Run standards in triplicate. Using 100-fold dilutions, generate a 5-point standard curve. We recommend running this several times and averaging data to generate a master standard curve.
3. Use the standard as the template and run a negative-strand real-time PCR reaction. Correlate Ct values to absolute fg amounts (Fig. 3).

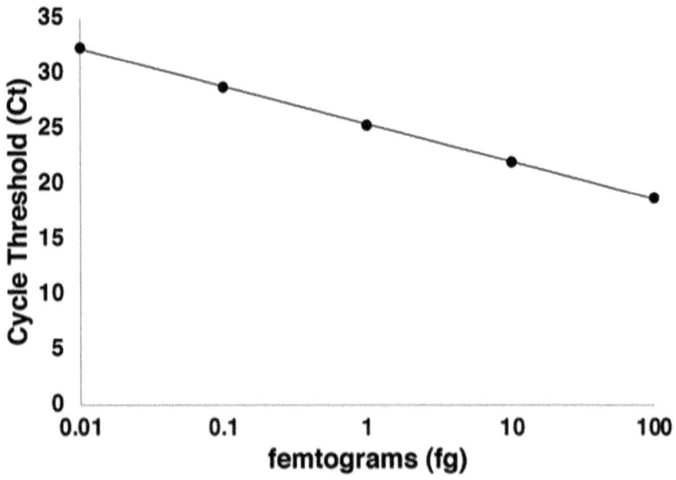

Fig. 3 Negative RV-16 real-time PCR standard curve. Serial dilutions of a synthetic negative-strand amplicon were used as a template and run in the negative-strand rhinovirus real-time PCR assay. The equation of the line is: $y = -1.475\ln(x) + 25.434$. Data are mean ± SEM ($n = 5$)

Convert average Ct values to fg using the equation of the line in Fig. 3:

$y = -1.475\ln(x) + 25.434$, solve for x.

$y = Ct$.

$x =$ sample fg value.

Absolute amounts can be converted to copy number as follows*:

Copy number = (Sample fg value $\times 6.022 \times 10^{23}$)/(79 bp $\times$ 660 g/mol $\times 1 \times 10^{15}$).

Avogadro's number $= 6.022 \times 10^{23}$.

Amplicon size = 79 bp.

Molecular weight of DNA = 660 g/mol.

*This is a base calculation. If determining the copy number from the initial sample is desired, then you would multiply the copy number by the RNA concentration for that sample as well as factor in all the dilutions you made during the RNA isolation, cDNA generation, and real-time PCR steps.

4 Notes

1. We expose epithelial cells to between $10^{4.5}$ and $10^{5.5}$ $TCID_{50}$ U/mL (correlating to a multiplicity of infection between ~0.1 and 1) of rhinovirus-16. In general, we use a lower infectious dose for cell lines and the higher dose for primary epithelial cells. Time of viral exposure and dose can be tailored to the cell type being used.

   The brief exposure with virus onto epithelial cells allows for binding and internalization. After washing the initial inoculum of virus away, the virus detected in the supernatant will be from actively replicating virus, which was released into the medium. The amount of internalized virus can also be determined.
2. We routinely use a 24-h post-infection time point, but this can be adjusted to other time points.
3. We have used many different methods for isolating intracellular RNA, such as TRIzol and commercially available column-based RNA isolation kits, with success. Guanidinium thiocyanate is a common chaotropic agent used in RNA lysis solution because it effectively lyses cells, denatures proteins, and inactivates RNases, thereby stabilizing nucleic acids. It is very important to lyse your cells immediately in RNA lysis buffer to avoid nonspecific degradation of nucleic acids in your sample and to maintain RNA integrity. Use standard best practices when working with RNA, which include wearing gloves, decontaminating your bench and equipment of RNases, and using RNase/DNase-free pipet tips and tubes. RNA should be treated with DNase to minimize possible genomic DNA contamination in your sample.

4. We have utilized various standard cDNA synthesis kits over the years with success, such as Superscript II (Invitrogen), Superscript III (Invitrogen), and 5X All-In-One MasterMix (Diamed).
5. Maxima Reverse Transcriptase is a reverse transcriptase that possesses RNase H activity. The RNase H activity cleaves the RNA strand of the RNA-DNA duplex. This ensures that there will be no RNA carry over into the real-time PCR reaction.
6. This primer contains a 5′ non-viral sequence from *Escherichia coli* combined with an RV-specific sequence to create a chimeric primer that avoids the phenomenon of self-priming. Self-priming is a common problem in the detection and quantification of many viruses and eliminates the ability for strand-specific detection.
7. Manufacturer's protocol suggests incubating at 50 °C, but we have shown that the specificity of this reaction increases with the higher temperature of 65 °C.

References

1. Leigh R, Proud D (2015) Virus-induced modulation of lower airway diseases: pathogenesis and pharmacologic approaches to treatment. Pharmacol Ther 148:185–198
2. Bochkov YA, Gern JE (2012) Clinical and molecular features of human rhinovirus C. Microbes Infect 14:484–494
3. van der Linden L, Wolthers KC, van Kuppeveld FLM (2015) Replication and inhibitors of enteroviruses and perechoviruses. Viruses 7: 4529–4562
4. Takeuchi O, Akira S (2009) Innate immunity to virus infection. Immunol Rev 227:75–86
5. Schönborn J, Oberstraß J, Breyel E, Tittgen J, Schumacher J, Lukacs N (1991) Monoclonal antibodies to double-stranded RNA as probes of RNA structure in crude nucleic acid extracts. Nucleic Acids Res 19:2993–3000
6. Warner SM, Wiehler S, Michi AN, Proud D (2019) Rhinovirus replication and innate immunity in highly differentiated human airway epithelial cells. Respir Res 20:150
7. Wiehler S, Proud D (2021) Specific assay of negative strand template to quantify intracellular levels of rhinovirus double-stranded RNA. Methods Protoc 4:13
8. Leigh R, Oyelusi W, Wiehler S, Koetzler R, Zaheer RS, Newton R, Proud D (2008) Human rhinovirus infection enhances airway epithelial cell production of growth factors involved in airway remodeling. J Allergy Clin Immunol 121:1238–1245
9. Lanford RE, Sureau C, Jacob JR, White R, Fuerst TR (1994) Demonstration of *in vitro* infection of chimpanzee hepatocytes with hepatitis C virus using strand-specific RT/PCR. Virology 202:606–614
10. Tuiskunen A, Leparc-Goffert I, Boubis L, Monteil V, Klingström J, Tolou HJ, Lundkvist A, Plumet S (2010) Self-priming of reverse transcriptase impairs strand-specific detection of dengue virus RNA. J Gen Virol 91:1017–1027
11. Vashist S, Urena L, Goodfellow I (2012) Development of a strand specific real-time RT-qPCR assay for the detection and quantification of murine norovirus RNA. J Virol Methods 184:69–76

Chapter 6

Determination of Binding and Endocytosis of Rhinovirus by Flow Cytometry

Umadevi Sajjan

Abstract

Viruses are dependent on their host cells for replication. The first step in viral infection is the binding of the virus to the host cell membrane, followed by internalization or endocytosis of the virus. Rhinoviruses utilize several cellular membrane receptors to cross the plasma membrane by endocytosis. Three major glycoprotein receptors that are utilized by rhinoviruses to gain entry into the cells are intracellular adhesion molecules, low-density lipoprotein receptor family members, and cadherin-related family member-3. Rhinovirus is endocytosed by a clathrin- or dynamin-dependent mechanism. Upon uptake into an acidic endosomal environment, rhinovirus uncoats and injects its genome into the cytoplasm, where the viral replication begins. It is often difficult to differentiate between bound and the endocytosed rhinovirus in the cells. Here, we describe a method to quantify bound and endocytosed virus by flow cytometry.

Key words Endosomes, Rhinovirus antibody, Immunofluorescence

1 Introduction

The first step in viral infection is the binding and entry of virus into the cell. Rhinoviruses are non-enveloped viruses and gain entry into host cells by receptor-mediated endocytosis. Rhinoviruses (RV) are classified into three species, RV-A, RV-B, and RV-C, which include more than 160 species. The majority of RV-A and RV-B species bind to human ICAM-1 [1]. Some RV-A species bind to the low-density lipoprotein receptor (LDLR) family, including very-LDLR and LDLR-related protein-1 [2, 3]. The receptor for RV-C was identified much later, and it binds to cadherin-related family 3 (CDHR3) [4]. Both RV-A and RV-B have been extensively studied and have been shown to enter cells via clathrin- or dynamin-dependent endocytosis [5, 6]. All the studies are conducted mostly in rhinovirus permissive HeLa cells, and the mechanism of entry may be dependent on the cell type [5]. Not much is known with regard to the entry or viral life cycle for RV-C due to

Umadevi Sajjan (ed.), *Rhinovirus: Methods and Protocols*, Methods in Molecular Biology, vol. 2903,
https://doi.org/10.1007/978-1-0716-4410-2_6,

limitations in the propagation of this virus. It is speculated that RV-C may hijack the host endocytic pathway similar to RV-A and RV-B after its binding to CDHR3.

Viruses stimulate distinct host signaling pathways at each step of the viral life cycle and may depend on the cell type. Airway epithelial cells lining the proximal airways are the primary target for all rhinoviruses. In airway epithelial cells, we showed that RV-A stimulates IL-8 via PI-3 kinase signaling, which coincides with endocytosis [7]. Rhinovirus binding to its receptors and recognition of double-stranded RNA generated during viral genome replication can also stimulate IL-8. To differentiate between the bound and internalized RV in HeLa cells and airway epithelial cell line, [^{35}S]-labeled RV was used [7, 8] in our previous study, which requires the use of radioactivity. Here we describe a flow cytometry method to differentiate between bound and internalized RV. This method encompasses using two different antibodies to rhinovirus and markers for early endosome and late endosome/lysosome markers Rab5 and Lamp1, respectively.

2 Materials

1. Bronchial epithelial cell line 16 HBE140 cells (Sigma Aldrich Cat# SCC150).
2. Rhinovirus RV-16 (ATCC). Propagate and purify the virus in H1HeLa cells as described in Chapter 2.
3. Type I bovine collagen (PureCol, Advanced Biomatrix Cat# 05005).
4. Minimum essential medium.
5. Heat-inactivated Fetal Bovine Serum.
6. Trypsin/EDTA.
7. Cell dissociation buffer (ThermoFisher Scientific, Cat# 13151014).
8. Sterile PBS with $CaCl_2$ and $MgCl_2$ (Gibco).
9. Rhinovirus VP2 antibody (QED Bioscience Cat# 18758).
10. Rhinovirus VP3 antibody (ThermoFisher Scientific Cat# MA5–18249).
11. Zenon™ Mouse IgG1 labelling kit with Alexa Fluor 647 (ThermoFisher Scientific Cat# Z25008).
12. Zenon™ Mouse IgG1 labelling kit with Alexa Fluor 488 (ThermoFisher Scientific Cat# Z25002).
13. APC-conjugated Rab5 antibody (Abcam Cat# an302988).
14. BD605-conjugated LAMP-1 (CD107α, BD biosciences Cat# 569302).

15. Zombie UV™ Fixable Viability Kit (BioLegend Cat# 423107).
16. Human Fc block (BD Biosciences Cat# 564219).
17. BD Cytofix/Cytoperm™ kit (BD Biosciences Cat# 554714).
18. Compensation beads (BioLegend, Cat# 424601).
19. Blocking buffer: 100 μL of MEM containing 1% serum, 0.02% sodium azide, 1× human FC block.
20. Cell culture incubator set at 37 °C.
21. Flow cytometer—Symphony (BD Biosciences) or similar.

3 Methods

3.1 Preparation of Labelled Antibodies

1. Mix 1 μg of VP2 or VP3 antibody in 20 μL of PBS with 5 μL of Zenon™ mouse IgG labelling reagent.
2. Use AlexaFluor 488 for VP2 and AlexaFluor 594 for VP3.
3. Incubate the mixture for 5 min at room temperature.
4. Add 5 μL of the Zenon™ blocking reagent to the reaction mixture.
5. Incubate the mixture for 5 min at room temperature. Store the labeled antibody at 4 °C.

3.2 Cell Culture and Infection

1. Coating of cell culture dishes with PureCol. Coat 10 cm and 6-well plates with PureCol (1 μg/cm$^{2.}$) for 16–18 h at 4 °C. Remove the unbound collagen and dry the plates under UV.
2. Complete medium: MEM + 10% heat-inactive fetal bovine serum +10% L-glutamine.
3. Serum-free medium: MEM + 10% L-glutamine.
4. Thaw a frozen vial of 16HBE140- cells in a 37 °C water bath.
5. Sterilize the outside of the vial with 70% ethanol and transfer the vial to the cell culture hood.
6. Transfer the cells from the vials to a 15 mL centrifuge tube containing 10 mL of warm medium. Invert gently two times to mix the content.
7. Centrifuge for 5 min at 500× *g*, 4 °C, and remove the supernatant by aspiration.
8. Resuspend the cell pellet in 1 mL of complete medium and transfer it to a collagen-coated 10-cm cell culture dish containing 10 mL of complete medium. Rotate the dish to evenly distribute the cells.
9. Incubate the cell culture dish in a cell culture incubator at 37 °C. Change the medium every 2 days.

10. When the cells reach 70–80% confluency, aspirate the medium and rinse the plate 2 times with 10 mL PBS without $CaCl_2$ and $MgCl_2$.
11. Add 3 mL of trypsin/EDTA and place it in an incubator for up to 2 min.
12. Tap the plate gently against the palm to release the adherent cells.
13. Centrifuge for 5 min at 500× *g*, 4 °C, and remove supernatant by aspiration.
14. Resuspend cell pellet in 5 mL of complete medium by pipetting up and down.
15. Count the cells using a cell counter or hemacytometer and suspend the cells in a complete medium to adjust the cell density to 1–3 × 10^6 cell/mL.
16. Plate the cells in three 6-well plates at a density of 5 × 10^5 cells/well and incubate for 24 h in a cell culture incubator.
17. Replace the medium with serum-free medium and continue to incubate for another 24 h.
18. Aspirate the medium and infect 3 wells in each plate with RV16 at 5 MOI in 500 μL of serum-free medium and another 3 wells with equal volume of sham.
19. Incubate the RV-infected plates at 37 °C; one plate for 30 min, the second plate for 60 min and the third plate for 90 min.
20. Incubate sham-infected cells for 90 min at 37 °C.

3.3 Staining of RV Bound to Cells

1. Perform all the centrifugation steps at 500×*g* for 5 min at 4 °C.
2. After incubating the cells with sham or RV as stated in **steps 19** and **20** of Subheading 3.2, aspirate the infection medium, rinse the cells with D-PBS twice.
3. Add 1 mL of cell dissociation buffer to each well and incubate for 5–10 min until the cells round up (*see* **Note 1**).
4. Gently tap the plate and collect the cells along with the dissociation buffer in 15 mL sterile conical tubes. Rinse the wells with 2 mL D-PBS to collect the remaining cells and combine them with the collected cell suspension.
5. Centrifuge, aspirate the supernatant, and suspend the cells in 2 mL of ice-cold PBS.
6. Repeat the centrifugation and suspend the cells in 100 μL of ice-cold PBS. Add 1 ul of 1:10 diluted UV-Zombie and incubate on ice for 15 min on ice in dark (*see* **Note 2**).
7. Add 2 mL of cold PBS and centrifuge.
8. Suspend the cell pellet in 100 μL of blocking buffer and incubate for 15 min on ice.

9. Add 10 μL of blocking buffer containing 0.5 μg of AlexaFluor 488-labeled anti-VP2 antibody and incubate for 30 min on ice.
10. Add 2 mL of ice-cold D-PBS and centrifuge.

3.4 Staining of Intracellular RV and Endosomes

1. Suspend cells from **step 10** of Subheading 3.2 in fixation and permeabilization buffer for 15 min on ice (*see* **Note 3**).
2. Add 2 mL of cold PBS and centrifuge.
3. Repeat washing with ice-cold D-PBS one more time.
3. Suspend cells in blocking buffer and add a mixture of VP3 (0.5 μg), Rab5, and LAMP-1 (according to the manufacturer's instructions) antibodies and incubate for 30 min on ice.
4. Add 2 mL of ice-cold D-PBS and centrifuge.
5. Suspend the cells in cold PBS for analysis by flow cytometry.
6. Pass the cells through a 70 μ filter to remove aggregated cells prior to analysis of cells by flow cytometry.

3.5 Controls for Flow Cytometry

1. These controls will be used for gating the cells.
2. Combine the cells from sham-infected cells after detachment of the cells from the 6-well plate.
3. Divide into 6 aliquots.
4. *Aliquot 1*: fix/permeabilize, wash the cells in cold PBS, and this is an unstained control.
5. *Aliquot 2*: Incubate the cells at 70 °C to kill the cells. Stain with UV-Zombie, fix/permeabilize, and wash the cells in cold PBS, and this is used as a control to remove the dead cells by gating after flow analysis (*see* **Note 4**).
6. *Aliquot 3*: Process the cells as described in Subheading 3.3, but do not add AlexaFluor 488-labeled RV16 antibody. Then continue the processing of cells as described in Subheading 3.4 to stain with intracellular RV and endosome markers, Rab5 and LAMP-1 antibodies. This is fluorescence minus one (FMO) control 1 (*see* **Note 5**).
7. *Aliquot 4, 5, and 6*: Process the cells as described in Subheading 3.3. Fix/permeabilize the cells as described in Subheading 3.4. Incubate aliquot 4 with VP3 and Rab5, aliquot 5 with VP3 and LAMP-1, and aliquot 6 with Rab5 and LAMP-1 antibodies. These will be FMO controls 2, 3, and 4.

3.6 Preparation of Compensation Controls

1. The compensation bead controls are used for adjusting the laser intensity in the flow cytometer and also for compensation so that there is no spillover from one channel to another.
2. Vortex compensation beads vigorously prior to using them to disrupt aggregates.

3. Prepare 4 tubes, one for each antibody (single color).
4. Add one drop of beads from each bottle (positive and negative).
5. Add the same concentration of antibody that is used for staining the cells, one antibody per tube.
6. Mix and incubate at room temperature for 15–20 min, protecting from exposure to light.
7. Add 2 mL D-PBS, centrifuge, and resuspend beads in D-PBS, and now they are ready for flow analysis.

3.7 Analysis of Cells by Flow Cytometry

1. Using the unstained cells, adjust the voltage in the forward and side scatter channel so that the cells are visible in the window (Fig. 1).
2. Analyze all the compensation beads to adjust the voltage for each fluorophore and to set the compensation (Fig. 2).
3. Analyze the dead cells stained with Zombie-UV to gate out the dead cells.
4. Then analyze all the FMO controls and the samples.

3.8 Analysis of the Samples by FlowJo Software

1. Transfer FCS files to FlowJo software.
2. Open the compensation matrix and confirm that the compensation is successful (Figs. 3 and 4).
3. Apply the compensation to all the samples and FMO controls.

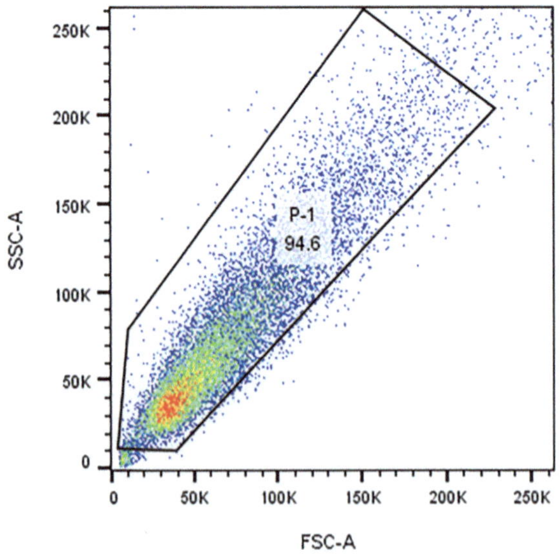

Fig. 1 Voltage adjusted in both SSC-A and FSC-A to obtain all the cells in the window. This is an important step. The P-1 gate is used to select the cells and exclude the cell debris

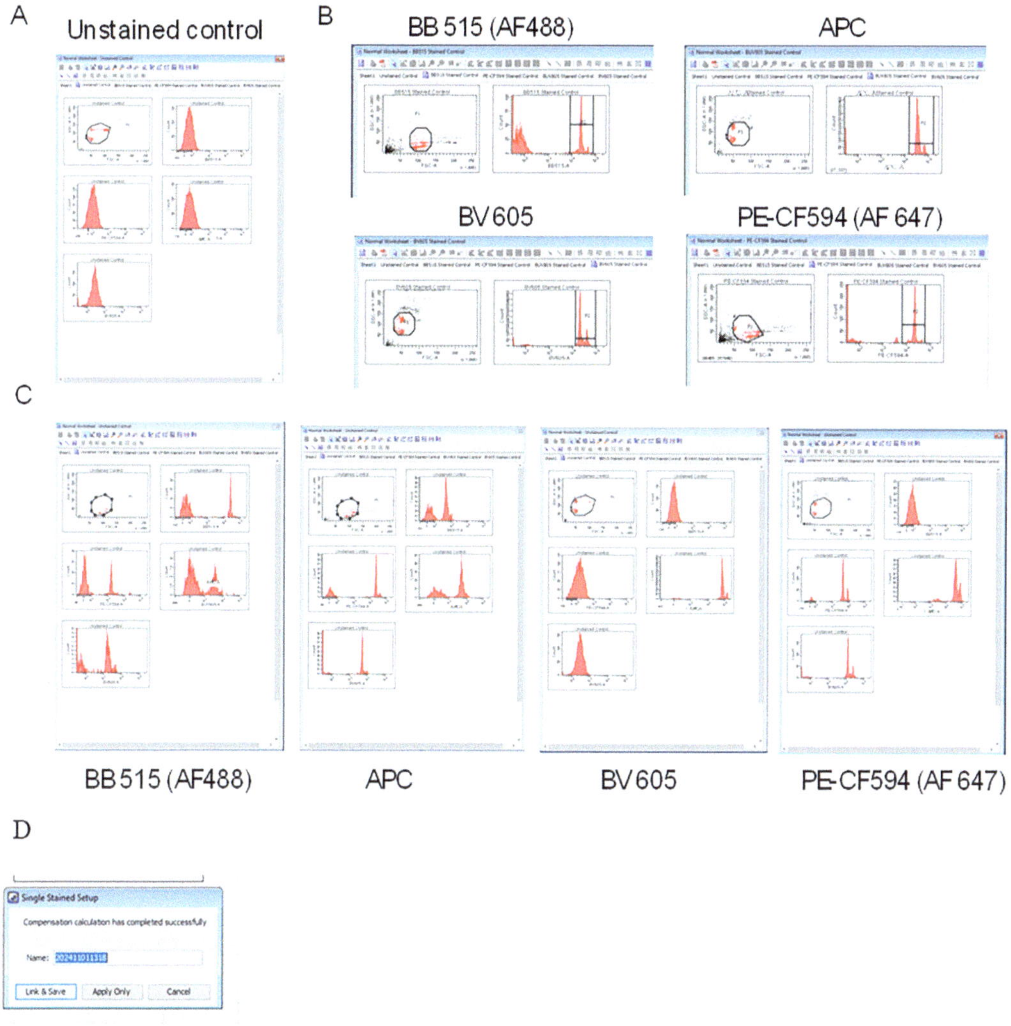

Fig. 2 Compensation using beads stained with a single fluorophore. (**a**) Unstained beads are used to gate the beads. (**b**) Beads stained with a single antibody are then run on the flow machine to adjust the voltage so that the peak for that specific fluorophore is well separated from the negative peak. (**c**) The voltage for each peak is adjusted to prevent the overlap of emission. The overlap is visualized for each fluorophore at the same time in the same window. (**d**) Indicates successful compensation. The successful compensation is extremely important prior to running actual samples

4. Using a sample which will supposedly be positive for all the antibodies should be analyzed first to apply appropriate gates using FMO controls.
5. Open RV-infected cells were incubated for 60 min for analysis. Apply P-1 gate to select the cells without debris (Fig. 5a).
6. Gate the cells using FSC-A vs. FSC-H to select single cells and remove doublets (Fig. 5b).

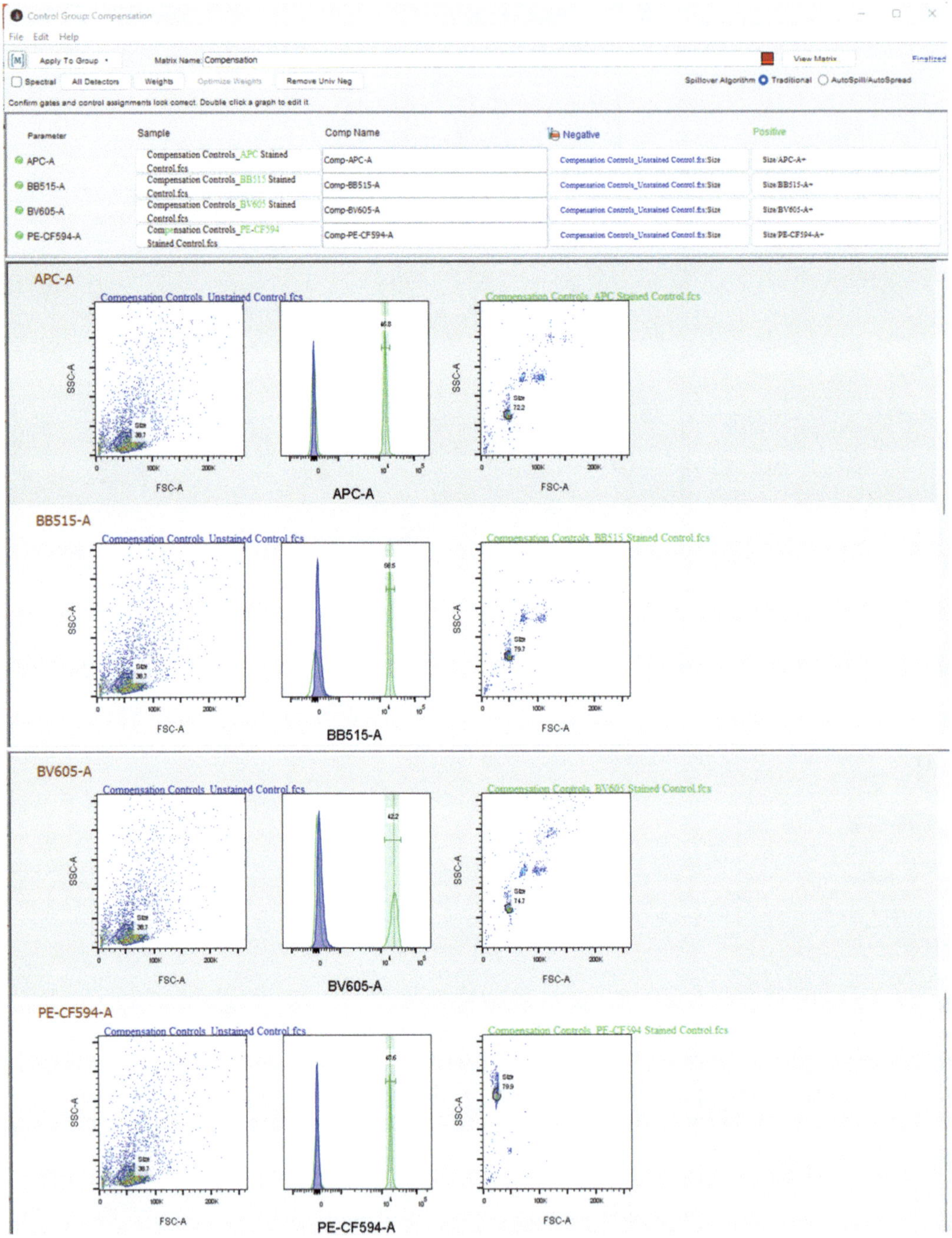

Fig. 3 Compensation matrix in the FlowJo analysis software. Compensation was examined in FlowJo. The green dots in the left of the upper panel indicate that the compensation calculations are correct. The bottom panel containing histograms shows the negative and positive peaks for each fluorophore

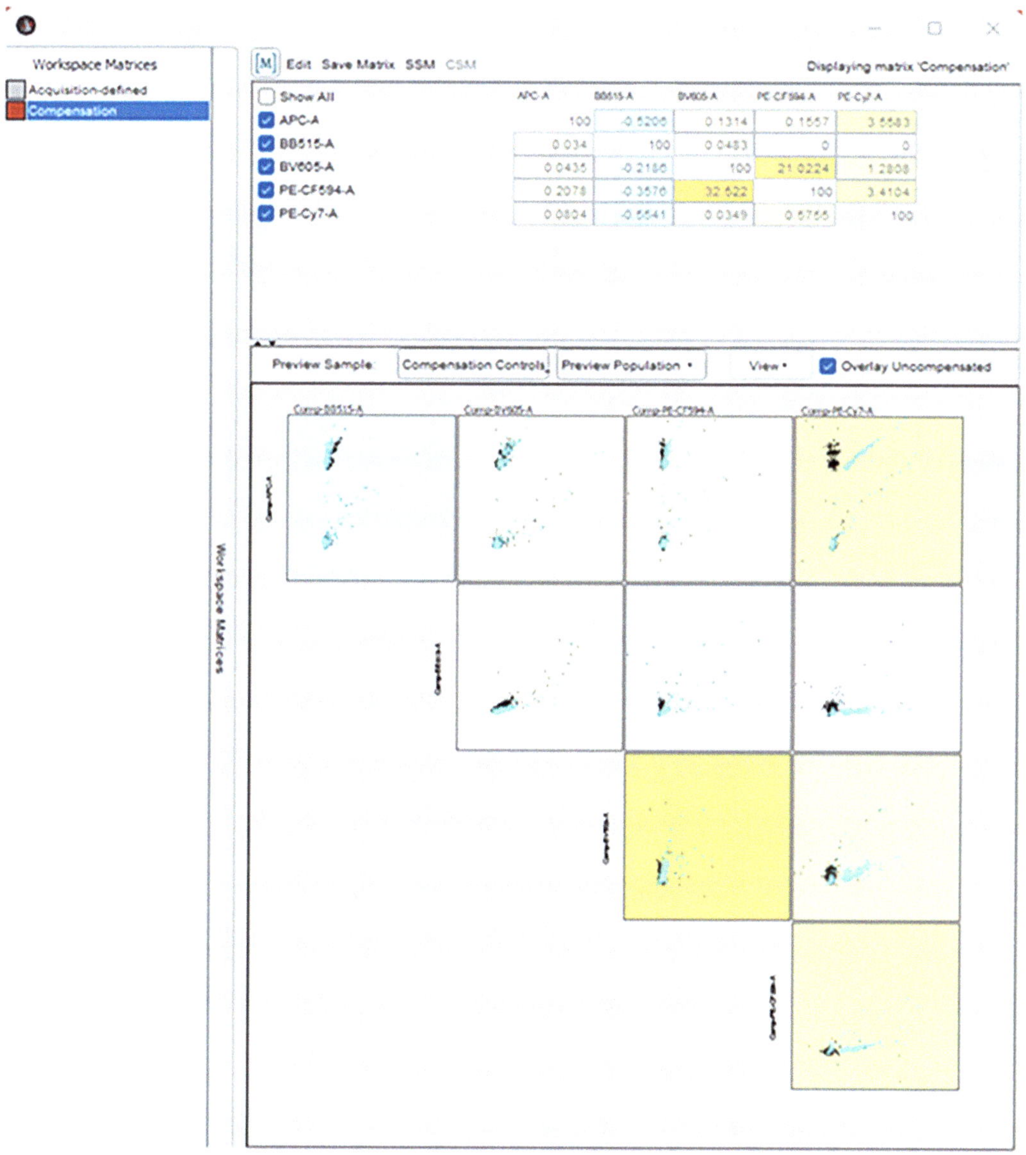

Fig. 4 The compensation matrix created by FlowJo. The compensation matrix generated in the FlowJo shows the compensation calculations applied for each color in the table to prevent non-specificity due to spillover from other channels. The bottom panel shows the compensation of each color. Black dots represent compensated matrix, and blue dots represent uncompensated matrix

7. Gate cells on Zombie gate to remove dead cells and select only live cells for further analysis (Fig. 5c).
8. It is important to remove cell debris, and the dead cells before analysis of cells to prevent non-specific staining and doublets to avoid overestimating the number of cells being positive for markers of interest.

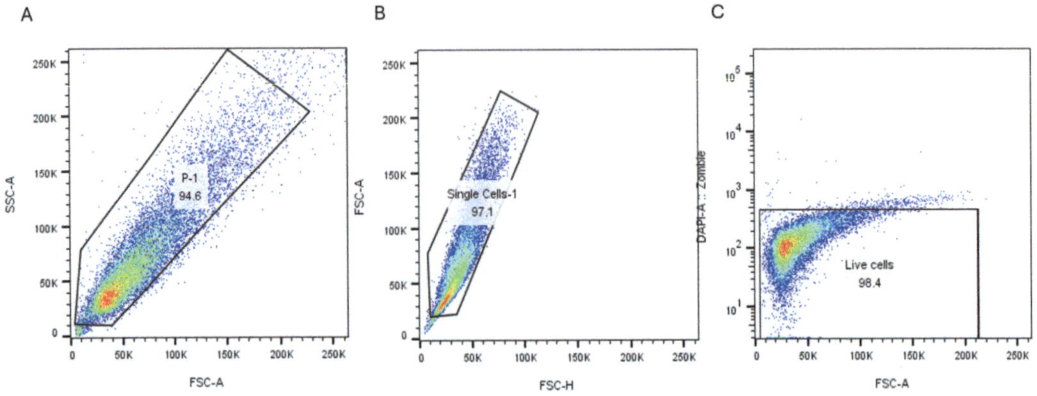

Fig. 5 Initial gating of the cells. Compensation matrix was applied to all the samples and the FMO control. Voltage of the side scatter and forward scatter channels was adjusted to capture majority of the cells. (**a**) The P-1 was applied to exclude the debris and aggregated cells. (**b**) The cells were then gated to remove doublets. (**c**) The cells were then gated based on the Zombie staining to remove the dead cells. The dead cells will be positive for Zombie

9. Gate positively stained live cells based on the specific FMO controls (Fig. 6).
10. Cells detected by VP2 antibody conjugated with AF 488 (comp-BB515-A) represent cells with bound RV.
11. Cells detected by VP3 antibody conjugated with AF 647 (comp-PE-CF294-A) represent cells with intracellular RV.
12. Cells detected by both VP2 and VP3 antibodies represent cells with both bound and intracellular RV.
13. All three populations of cells that were positive for RV were further analyzed for the presence of early endosomes (Rab5 APC) and late endosomes (LAMP-1, BV604).
14. Sham-infected cells were neither positive for bound RV nor for intracellular RV (Fig. 6a).
15. Cells incubated with RV for 30 min showed primarily bound RV, but not internalized RV (Fig. 6b).
16. Cells incubated with RV for 60 min showed cell populations that were positive for bound RV, internalized RV, and both bound and internalized RV (Fig. 6c).
17. Cells incubated with RV for 90 min showed cell populations that were positive for bound RV, internalized RV and both bound and internalized RV, with the majority of the cells being positive for internalized RV (Fig. 6d).
18. The data from all three replicates were used to determine the % of live cells positive for c (Table 1).
19. One of the samples that is cells infected with RV and incubated for 60 min was further analyzed for the expression of Rab5 (APC) and LAMP-1 (BV 604).

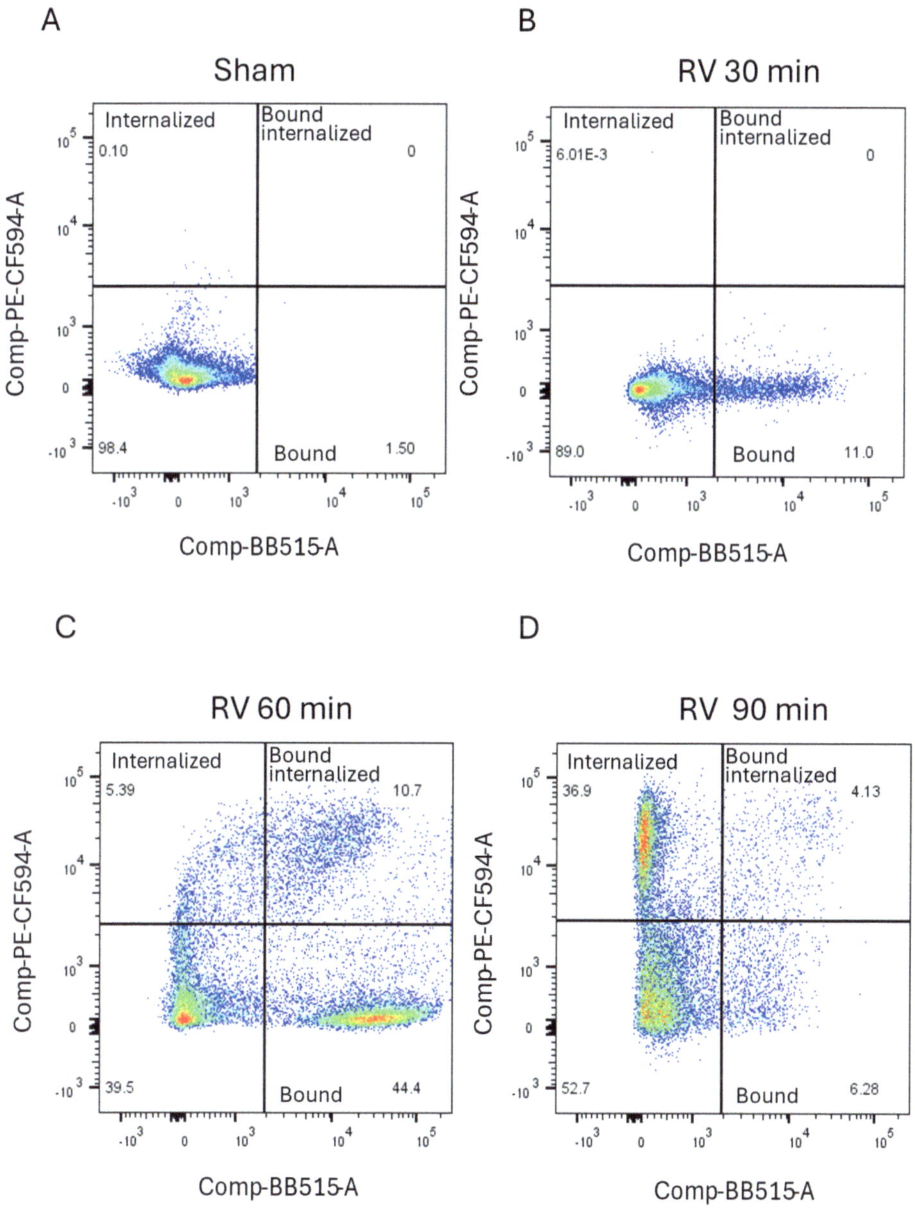

Fig. 6 Analysis of cells by FlowJo. Live cells were gated for positivity with AF 488 (Comp-B515-A, represents cells with bound RV) and AF 647 (Comp-PE-CF594-A, represents cells with internalized RV) using appropriate FMO controls. By this gating we identified four populations. Cells with no bound or internalized RV (bottom left quadrangle), cells with bound RV (bottom right quadrangle), cells with internalized RV (upper left quadrangle), and cells with both bound and internalized RV (upper right quadrangle)

Table 1
Quantification of cells with bound, internalized, and bound/internalized RV by flow cytometry

Infection	Time (min)	Bound RV	Bound/internalized RV	Internalized RV
Sham	90	0.00	0.00	0.00
RV	30	12.73 ± 2.80	1.13 ± 0.54	0.03 ± 0.06
RV	60	39.2 ± 4.65	13.24 ± 2.71	7.03 ± 1.56
RV	90	10.74 ± 4.48	5030 ± 1.98	36.7 ± 6.10

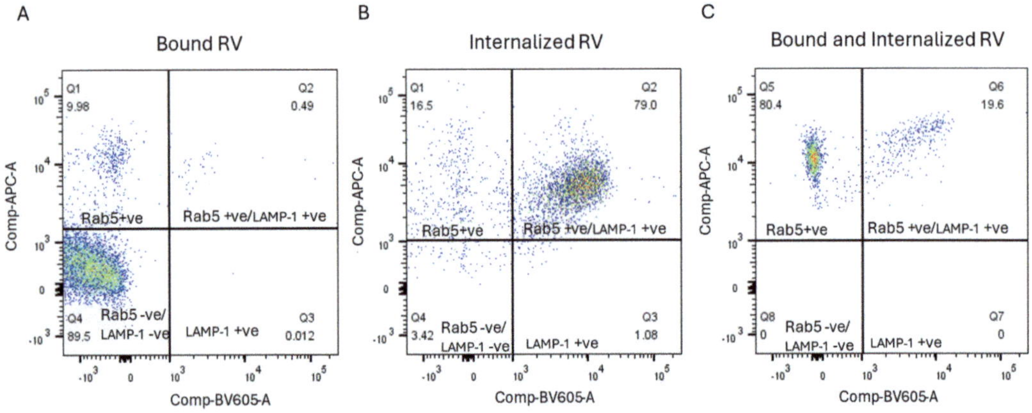

Fig. 7 Analysis of cells positive for bound, internalized, and a mixture of bound and internalized RV (AF 647). Cells infected with RV and incubated for 60 min were first gated on VP2 and VP3 antibodies. Cell populations positive for bound, internalized, and both bound and internalized RV were further gated on Rab5 (Comp-APC-A) and LAMP1 (Comp-BV605-A)

20. Each population of cells, that is, cells with bound RV, internalized RV, and both bound and internalized RV, were analyzed separately for the expression of Rab5 (APC) and LAMP-1 (BV 604) (Fig. 7).
21. Cells with bound, and bound and internalized RV showed more early endosomes than late endosomes.
22. Cells with only internalized RV showed more late endosomes than early endosomes. This may be due to endosomes containing RV maturing to late endosomes, when the pH of the endosomes becomes more acidic. This is necessary for internalized RV to inject their genome into the cytoplasm, a necessary step in the viral replication (*see* **Note 6**).

4 Notes

1. If the cells don't come off of the plate, gently pipette the dissociation buffer on the attached cells with 1 mL pipetteman to release the cells.
2. The UV-Zombie positive cells were excluded during the analysis. The dead cells have compromised plasma membrane, therefore the antibody used for detection of cell surface RV can potentially detect the intracellular endocytosed RV.
3. After fixation and permeabilization the cells can be stored at 4 ° C overnight.
4. The heat-killed cells will stain with UV-Zombie and are used to detect the gating out the dead cells during analysis by flow cytometry.
5. The unstained control, cells stained with Zombie alone and FMO controls are extremely important to gate the positive cells for each fluorophore and to avoid the signals spilling from other channels.
6. Please note that this assay will not indicate whether the internalized RV is present in early or later endosomes. It only indicates an increase in endosomes and late endosomes.

References

1. Uncapher CR, DeWitt CM, Colonno RJ (1991) The major and minor group receptor families contain all but one human rhinovirus serotype. Virology 180:814–817
2. Hofer F, Gruenberger M, Kowalski H, Machat H, Huettinger M, Kuechler E, Blaas D (1994) Members of the low density lipoprotein receptor family mediate cell entry of a minor-group common cold virus. Proc Natl Acad Sci USA 91:1839–1842
3. Marlovits TC, Abrahamsberg C, Blaas D (1998) Very-low-density lipoprotein receptor fragment shed from HeLa cells inhibits human rhinovirus infection. J Virol 72:10246–10250
4. Bochkov YA, Watters K, Ashraf S, Griggs TF, Devries MK, Jackson DJ, Palmenberg AC, Gern JE (2015) Cadherin-related family member 3, a childhood asthma susceptibility gene product, mediates rhinovirus C binding and replication. Proc Natl Acad Sci USA 112:5485–5490
5. Fuchs R, Blaas D (2012) Productive entry pathways of human rhinoviruses. Adv Virol 2012: 826301
6. Snyers L, Zwickl H, Blaas D (2003) Human rhinovirus type 2 is internalized by clathrin-mediated endocytosis. J Virol 77:5360–5369
7. Newcomb DC, Sajjan U, Nanua S, Jia Y, Goldsmith AM, Bentley JK, Hershenson MB (2005) Phosphatidylinositol 3-kinase is required for rhinovirus-induced airway epithelial cell interleukin-8 expression. J Biol Chem 280: 36952–36961
8. Herdy B, Snyers L, Reithmayer M, Hinterdorfer P, Blaas D (2004) Identification of the human rhinovirus serotype 1A binding site on the murine low-density lipoprotein receptor by using human-mouse receptor chimeras. J Virol 78:6766–6774

Chapter 7

Assessment of Viral Replication in Rhinovirus-Infected Airway Epithelial Cells

Michelle E. Love, Shahina Wiehler, and David Proud

Abstract

The ability to titer virus is critical for quantifying the efficacy of interventions on viral replication as well as for monitoring the consistency and viability of viral stocks to ensure reproducible experiments. Infectious rhinovirus is quantified by determining the dilution of virus that infects and causes cytopathic effects in a permissive cell line. Here we outline a protocol for determining tissue culture infectious dose 50 ($TCID_{50}$) of rhinovirus-16 in WI-38 fibroblasts using an adapted microtiter plate system.

Key words Viral titer, Rhinovirus, WI-38 fibroblasts, Tissue Culture Infectious dose 50 ($TCID_{50}$), Microtiter plate

1 Introduction

Human rhinovirus (RV) infections are responsible for the majority of common colds and are also important triggers of exacerbations of lower airway diseases, such as asthma, chronic obstructive pulmonary disease, and cystic fibrosis [1]. The airway epithelial cell is the major site of RV infection [2, 3], but, in contrast to viruses such as influenza, RV does not cause overt cytotoxicity in epithelial cells either in vitro or in vivo [4–6]. Therefore, RV viral titers cannot be assayed using their natural host cell. Thus, over many years, various cell lines, usually of fibroblast origin, have been selected to monitor viral titers based on their susceptibility to RV-induced cytotoxicity. This is made more complex by the fact that different strains of RV and, indeed, even different clinical isolates of the same RV strain, may have different capacities to cause cytopathic effects in various cell lines depending upon the cell type that isolate has been "trained" to replicate in most efficiently. For example, among strains commonly used in our own laboratory, the isolate of the RV-1A strain we use replicates and causes cytotoxicity most effectively in H1HeLa cells, and so we use this cell line to titer our

Umadevi Sajjan (ed.), *Rhinovirus: Methods and Protocols*, Methods in Molecular Biology, vol. 2903,
https://doi.org/10.1007/978-1-0716-4410-2_7,

RV-1A. By contrast, the isolate of RV-16 that we use replicates most effectively in WI-38 cells. Thus, while the various steps we describe for our protocol for monitoring titers of RV-16 using WI-38 cells will remain largely unchanged for other strains, the reader must consider the cell type to be used to obtain the most effective response to the specific RV isolate of interest.

Conventionally, RV titers are expressed as the dose that causes lysis in 50% of samples (tubes or wells) of cells using standard calculation methods, such as those based on the Reed-Muench method [7]. Traditionally, monolayers of cells would be grown in roller tubes and infected with dilutions of virus. Cytopathic effects were determined by visual inspection after 5 days. This model is limited in that it is labor intensive and requires large numbers of tubes to provide accuracy. Additionally, the assessment of lysis by visual assessment is somewhat subjective and provides no objective record that can be saved for later inspection.

To overcome these limitations, the method described here has been adapted to use 96-well culture plates. Each of several serial dilutions of virus-containing samples is loaded into two columns of a 96-well plate, such that each dilution of virus is assayed in 16 replicates. Following an appropriate incubation period, the cells are fixed and stained with crystal violet, which is taken up by intact cells. Cytopathic effects result in a decrease in monolayer integrity and, therefore, a loss of staining that is detected as a reduction in absorbance at 570 nm using a microtiter plate reader. The dilution of sample that reduces monolayer integrity in 50% of replicate wells is used to calculate the tissue culture infectious dose 50 ($TCID_{50}$).

2 Materials

WI-38 cell culture medium.

1× MEM (+) Earle's Salts, (−) L-Glutamine

10% heat inactivated fetal bovine serum (FBS)

2 mM L-glutamine

100 U/mL penicillin streptomycin

1 mM sodium pyruvate

1× MEM non-essential amino acid solution

Store the prepared WI-38 cull culture medium at 4 °C. Warm the medium to 37 °C in a water bath prior to feeding cells.

F12 10% FBS.

1×F12 medium

10% heat inactivated fetal bovine serum (FBS)

Store prepared F12 10% FBS at 4 °C, warm the medium to 37 °C in a water bath before using on cells.

1× hanks buffered saline solution (HBSS)

1× TrypLE Select enzyme

Erythrosin B.

1× Piperazine-N,N′-bis(2-ethanesulfonic acid), (PIPES)

5% heat inactivated fetal bovine serum (FBS)

1.5 mg/mL Erythrosin B

Filter the solution and store at 4 °C for short-term use or in aliquots at −20 °C for long-term storage.

2% v/v Gluteraldehyde

Dulbecco's Phosphate buffered saline, (−) Ca^{2+}, (−) Mg^{2+}.

Gluteraldehyde is toxic; prepare this solution in a fume hood.

0.1% w/v crystal violet

Distilled water.

3 Methods

Titering rhinovirus in WI-38 fibroblasts consists of the following steps (Fig. 1):

1. Propagating WI-38 fibroblasts.
2. Splitting WI-38 fibroblasts.
3. Seeding 96-well plates.
4. Infecting cells with sample dilutions.
5. Staining plates.
6. Calculating viral titer.

3.1 Thawing WI-38 Cells

1. As noted above, we describe the methods for titering RV-16 in WI-38 fibroblasts, but the same steps can be applied for other applicable cell lines. WI-38 fibroblasts can either be used directly from frozen stock vials from ATCC, or each stock vial can be expanded and passaged to create stocks of passage 1 and passage 2 cells for titer. Expanded WI-38 cells are frozen down at a concentration of 2 × 10^6 cells/mL.
2. To expand cells for titer, thaw a single vial of either ATCC or passaged WI-38 into 10 mL of pre-warmed F12 with 10% FBS. Centrifuge the thawed cells at 125× *g* for 8 min at room temperature. Gently aspirate the supernatant and resuspend the cell pellet in 10 mL of WI-38 medium. The cell suspension is then transferred to a T175 flask containing 15 mL of WI-38 medium and incubated at 37 °C and 5% CO_2. Cells are fed with

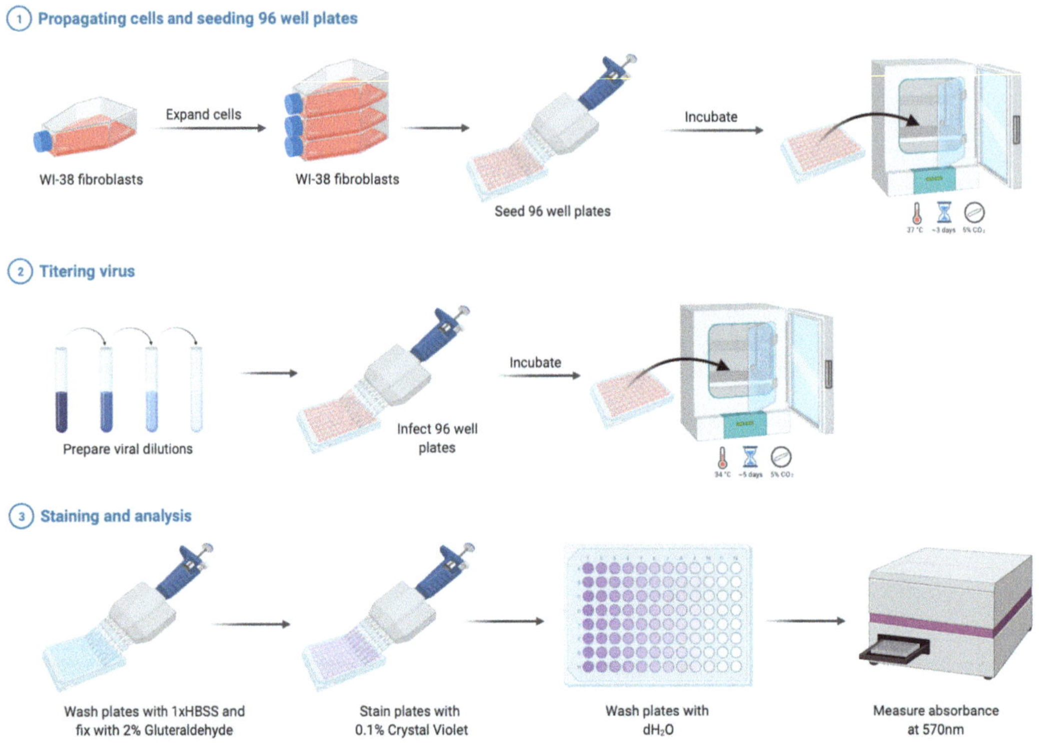

Fig. 1 Workflow for titering RV

25 mL of pre-warmed medium every 2–3 days until confluent (*see* **Note 1**).

3.2 Splitting WI-38 Fibroblasts

1. Depending on the number of samples to be titered, cells can be split and passaged into additional T175 flasks. Three 96-well plates are required for each sample to be titered. On average, one confluent T175 flask typically contains enough cells to seed six 96-well plates. Therefore, if titering two or fewer samples, you may skip this step and proceed to Subheading 3.3, Seeding 96-well plates.
2. To split cells, aspirate the medium from each flask and wash the cell monolayers with 15 mL warm 1xHBSS to remove residual WI-38 culture medium, since FBS contains inhibitors and proteins that reduce the efficacy of cell dissociation enzymes. Add 7 mL prewarmed TrypLE Select enzyme and incubate the flask at 37 °C until the cells are lifted. Cells lift very quickly, so it is important to check the flask frequently under the microscope. Gently tapping the flask can assist with the lifting process. While the cells are lifting, pipette 10 mL of prewarmed F12 medium containing 10% FBS into a sterile 50 mL conical tube. Once lifted, transfer the cell suspension to the sterile 50 mL tube containing the F12/10% FBS combination.

Rinse the flask with an additional 10 mL of F12 medium containing 10% FBS to recover any cells that may have been left behind and transfer this suspension to the same tube. Centrifuge the cell suspension at 125× *g* for 8 min at room temperature. When centrifugation is complete, aspirate the supernatant and resuspend the cell pellet in 10 mL of WI-38 medium. Transfer 20 μL of Erythrocin B to a 1.5 mL tube and add 20 μL of the cell suspension, gently pipetting up and down to mix. Load 20 μL of the Erythrocin B cell suspension mixture into a Neubauer hemocytometer. Count viable cells in at least two of the 4 × 4 grids. Counts should be within 10% of each other. If not, count additional grids until counts are close together. Calculate the average number of cells. Do not count cells that have stained red, as they are not viable. Calculate the total number of cells using the following calculation:

$$\text{Average number of cells in } 4 \times 4 \text{ grids} \times 2 \times 10{,}000 \times 10\ \text{mL} = \text{Total number of cells}$$

Seed the required number of T175 flasks by resuspending cells in 25 mL of cell culture media and transferring to new T175 flasks. WI-38 cells are seeded at a density of 2×10^6 cells per T175 flask. Return cells to the incubator set at 37 °C and 5% CO_2 and continue to feed every 2–3 days until confluent (*see* **Note 1**).

3.3 Seeding 96-Well Plates

1. To seed 96-well plates, lift cells from the required number of T175 flasks. To do this, aspirate the medium from each flask and wash the cell monolayers with 15 mL warm 1xHBSS. Add 7 mL prewarmed TrypLE Select enzyme per flask and incubate at 37 °C until the cells are lifted. Cells lift very quickly so make sure to check the flask frequently under the microscope. Gently tapping the flask can assist with the dissociation process. While the cells are incubating, pipette 10 mL of prewarmed F12 medium containing 10% FBS into a sterile 50 mL conical tube. Once lifted transfer the cell suspension to the tube containing the F12/10% FBS solution. Rinse the flask with an additional 10 mL F12 medium containing 10% FBS to recover any cells may have been left behind and transfer this suspension to the same conical tube. Centrifuge the cell suspension at 125× *g* for 8 min at room temperature. When centrifugation is complete aspirate off the supernatant and resuspend the cell pellet in 10 mL of WI-38 medium. Transfer 20 μL of Erythrosin B to a 1.5 mL microcentrifuge tube and add 20 μL of the cell suspension, gently pipetting up and down to mix. Load 20 μL of the Erythrosin B cell suspension mixture into a Neubauer hemocytometer. Count cells in at least two of the 4 × 4 grids and calculate the average number of cells. Do not

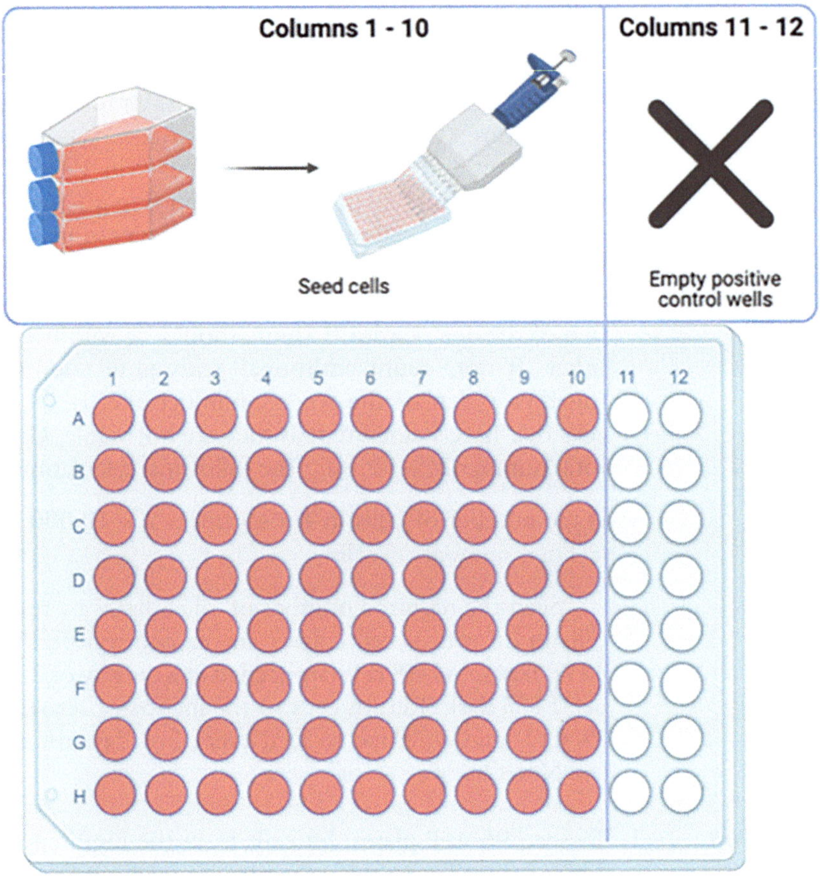

Fig. 2 Plate set up for seeding 96-well plates for titer. Empty wells in columns 11 and 12 do not contain cells and are used as a positive control for 100% lysis (minimum absorbance at 570 nm)

count cells that have stained red, as they are not viable. Calculate the total number of cells using the following calculation:

$$\text{Average number of cells in } 4 \times 4 \text{ grids} \times 2 \times 10{,}000 \times 10 \text{ mL} = \text{Total number of cells}$$

2. WI-38 cells are resuspended to a concentration of 8×10^5 cells/mL. Gently transfer the cell suspension to a sterile solution basin. Using a multichannel pipette, transfer 100 uL per well into columns 1 through 10 of the 96-well plate (*see* Fig. 2). Work quickly as cells rapidly fall out of solution; if multiple plates are to be loaded, it may be necessary to periodically pipette the solution up and down to resuspend the cells. Columns 11 and 12 of each plate are left empty; these wells will be used as a positive control for 100% lysis (minimum theoretical absorption) when the plates are stained (Fig. 2). Place the cells in an incubator set at 37 °C and 5% CO_2 and leave until the cells reach confluence, approximately 3 days (*see* **Note 2**).

3.4 Infecting Cells with Sample Dilutions

1. Serial dilutions of virus are calculated such that when 100 μL of sample is added to 100 μL of cell culture medium already in each well, the appropriate final dilution of sample is reached in each well at the final 200 μL (Fig. 3). WI-38 cells are incubated for 5 days with RV-16 samples, and therefore, we replace the medium prior to loading the viral dilutions (*see* **Note 3**). Each dilution of viral sample is loaded into two columns of a 96-well plate for a total of 16 replicates (Fig. 4). To replace the medium, tilt the plate and gently aspirate the medium out of each well; do not allow the aspirator to touch the cells growing at the bottom. Disruption of cell monolayers can trigger cell peeling and will result in a false positive well when the cells are stained.
2. We recommend that all samples collected from rhinovirus-infected human airway epithelial cells should be tested in dilutions ranging from 1:100 to 1:3,000,000. Perform half-log serial dilutions in cell culture media on each sample to be titered (Fig. 3). Make sure to vortex test tubes between each transfer to ensure thorough mixing of the virus in each sample. Once you have run this type of assay several times on the type of sample you are analyzing and get a better idea of the $TCID_{50}$ values you obtain, then it becomes possible to reduce the range of dilutions needed for each sample.
3. Pipette 100 μL of cell culture medium into the first two columns of each 96-well plate. No viral cell lysis will occur in these wells, so they will be used as the negative control when measuring absorbance (0% cell lysis, maximum absorbance). The last two columns of each plate are left empty and will be used as the positive control for each plate (100% cell lysis, minimum absorbance). Pipette 100 μL of each viral dilution into wells of duplicate columns as shown in Fig. 4. Transfer plates to an incubator set at 34 °C and 5% CO_2. Incubation times vary

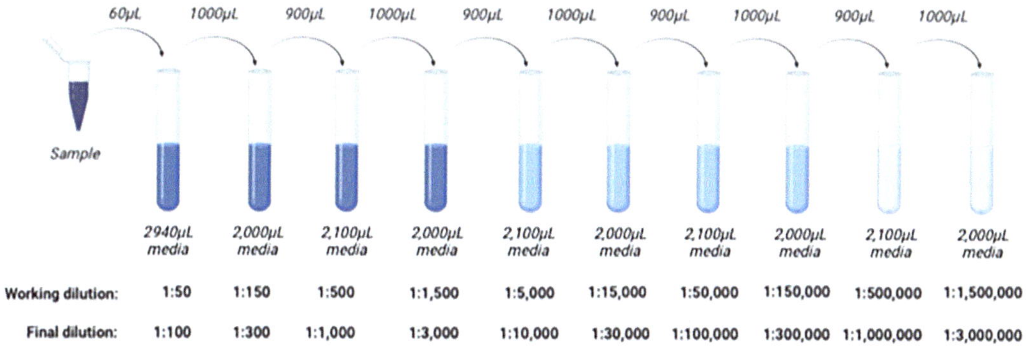

Fig. 3 Standard serial dilutions for titering rhinovirus

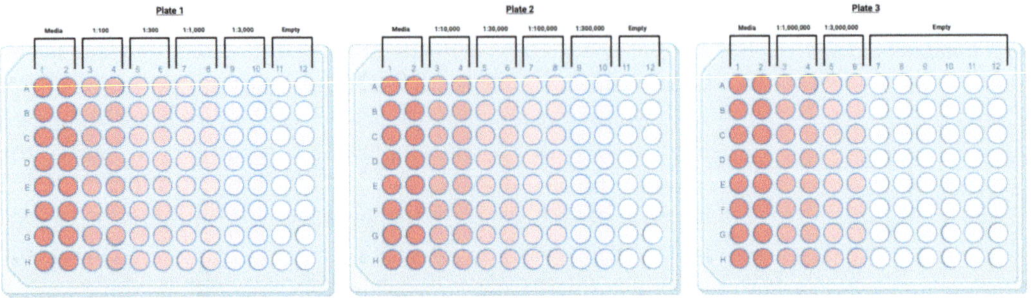

Fig. 4 Template for loading sample dilutions into 96-well plates

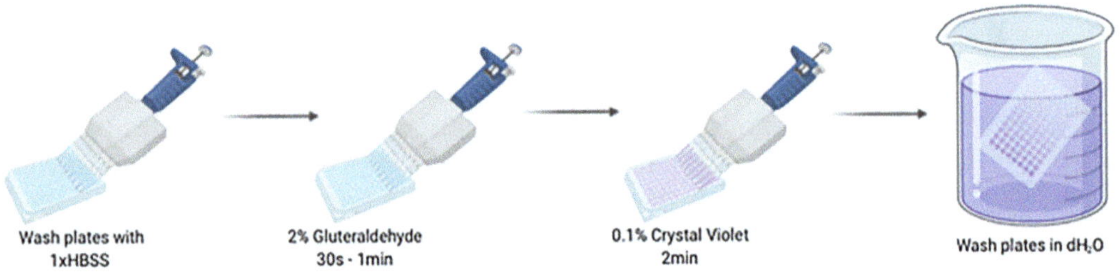

Fig. 5 Workflow for staining viral titer plates

depending on the cell line used. WI-38 cells are incubated for 5 days prior to staining.

3.5 Staining Viral Titer Plates

On the day of staining, prepare 2% Gluteraldehyde and 0.1% crystal violet. Carefully shake the media out of the 96-well plates into a suitable waste container. Use a multichannel pipette to add 100 μL of pre-warmed 1xHBSS (without Ca^{2+} or Mg^{2+}) into each well to wash the plates. Carefully shake out the 1xHBSS and add 100 μL per well 2% Gluteraldehyde for 30 s to 1 min to fix the cells. Gently shake out the 2% Gluteraldehyde and add 100 μL per well 0.1% crystal violet. Incubate the plates for 20 min at room temperature to stain. Once staining is complete, gently shake out the 0.1% crystal violet into a waste container. Fill a 4 L beaker with distilled water and submerge the plates to rinse; repeat three more times, each with fresh distilled water, until all the excess stain has been washed off the plates (Fig. 5). When washing is complete, shake any excess water out into the sink and allow plates to air dry upside down without lids on a pad of paper towels. This usually takes overnight. Once the plates have dried, clean the bottom surface of each plate with 70% ethanol to remove any residual crystal violet and measure absorbance at 570 nm using a microtiter plate reader.

3.6 Calculating Viral Titer

$TCID_{50}$ for each sample is calculated using the Reed-Muench method [7]. In the context of this assay, the dilution of virus that causes cytopathic effect reducing monolayer integrity and therefore absorbance in 50% of stained wells below a defined value is considered the 50% endpoint. To define a well that shows a cytopathic effect, we take the average absorbance of the 16 buffer wells (no lysis, maximum absorbance) and subtract the average absorbance of the 16 empty wells (100% lysis, minimum absorbance). We divide this value in half and add it back to the average value of the empty wells. (For example, if the buffer wells have an absorbance of 0.55 and the empty wells have an average absorbance of 0.05, the difference is 0.5. We divide 0.5 by 2 to get 0.25 and add back to the empty well absorbance to get a value of 0.3). We arbitrarily define all absorbance values below this calculated number as having a cytopathic effect, while those above this number are not significantly lysed. We acknowledge that this is an arbitrary definition, but it removes subjective assessments and gives an absolute number. It is important to note, however, that few individual wells demonstrate a precisely 50% reduction in absorbance; most wells are clearly above or below this level (*see* **Note 4**). To meet the 50% definition, at least 8 of the 16 replicate wells for a sample dilution must demonstrate a sufficient reduction in absorbance. For each sample dilution, tally the number of cytopathic wells and cumulative cytopathic wells across all the dilutions (*see* **Note 4**) and calculate the percentage cytopathic effect. See Table 1 for an example data table. Rarely will a given sample dilution equate exactly to the 50% endpoint. More often one dilution will be above, and one dilution will be below 50%, therefore it is necessary to calculate the proportionate distance between these dilutions. Proportionate distance is then used to calculate $TCID_{50}$ per unit volume using the formula below. Recall the sample dilution volume was 200 μL per well. For example, data and calculations, *see* Fig. 6 and **Note 5**.

Table 1
Example viral titer data

Log of virus dilution	Cytopathic wells	Cumulative cytopathic wells (A)	Cumulative non-cytopathic wells (B)	Ratio of A/(A + B)	Percent positive cytopathic (%)
−3	16/16	53	0	53/53	100
−3.5	16/16	37	0	37/37	100
−4	10/16	21	6	21/27	77.8
−4.5	7/16	11	15	11/26	42.3
−5	4/16	4	27	4/31	12.9
−5.5	0/16	0	43	0/43	0
−6	0/16	0	59	0/59	0
−6.5	0/16	0	75	0/75	0

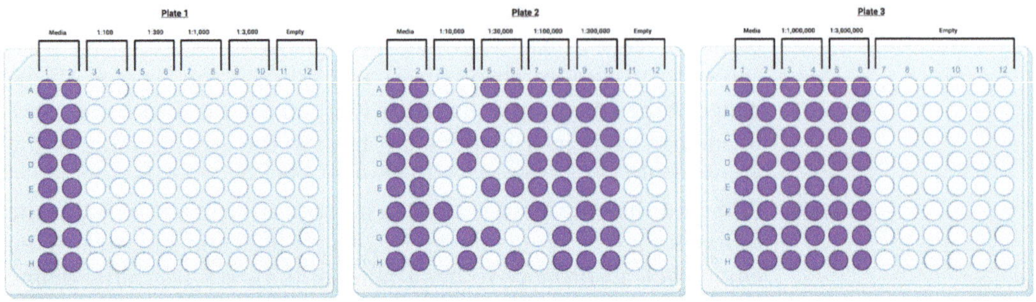

Fig. 6 Example data following crystal violet staining

$$\text{Proportionate distance} = \frac{(\%\text{positive above }50\%) - 50\%}{(\%\text{positive above }50\%) - (\%\text{positive below }50\%)}$$

$$\begin{aligned}\text{Log ID}_{50} = {} & (\text{Log dilution with} > 50\%\text{cytopathic}) \\ & + (\text{proportionate distance})(\text{Log dilution factor})\end{aligned}$$

$$\text{TCID}_{50}\text{ per }200\mu\text{L} = 10\text{ Log ID}_{50}$$

$$\text{TCID}_{50}\text{ per mL} = 5 \times 10\text{ Log ID}_{50}$$

4 Notes

1. WI-38 secretes growth factors that promote their own propagation. Therefore, when feeding WI-38 cells, remove only 12.5 mL of spent media from the T175 flask and replace it with 13 mL fresh cell culture media.
2. We have found WI-38 cells adhere and grow differently depending on the brand of plastic wear used. Grown on some plastics, these cells will exhibit peeling around the edges of wells after staining. If growing WI-38 cells for the first time in 96-well plates, we recommend testing growth on multiple plastic wear brands and determining the appropriate length of time for cells to reach 100% confluence before tittering samples. Other cell lines may vary in their affinity for plastic and growth time. For example, H1HeLa cells have a rapid doubling time; therefore, to minimize peeling, cells should be seeded at low density in 96-well plates and infected at sub-confluence.
3. Depending on the cell line used and the length of incubation, the cell culture medium may need to be replaced before loading viral dilutions.
4. Although we have established an absorbance value that must be below for a cytopathic effect in that well to be established, we still encourage the reader to visually examine each plate. It

must be remembered that the light beam of the microtiter plate reader is very narrow. Although rare, it is possible that a well may be almost completely lysed, but a small clump of cells may have survived in the middle of the well where the light beam passes. In this case the absorbance may not meet the requirements for the well to be defined as showing a cytopathic effect even though lysis has clearly occurred. By contrast, peeling or a small pinhole in the center of the well may lead to a "false positive." In each of these rare cases, therefore, it may be necessary to manually define the well as lysed or not in order to give an accurate value.

5. $TCID_{50}$ example calculation based on data in Fig. 6.

   Proportionate distance example calculation:

   Based on the data from Table 1, *the 50% endpoint lies somewhere between the* 10^{-4} *(77.8% cytopathic) and* $10^{-4.5}$ *(42.3% cytopathic) dilutions.*

$$\text{Proportionate distance} = \frac{77.8\% - 50\%}{77.8\% - 42.3\%} = 0.78$$

$$\text{Log ID}_{50} = (-4) + (0.78)(-0.5) = -4.39$$

$$\text{TCID}_{50} \text{ per } 200\ \mu\text{L} = 10^{4.39}$$

$$\text{TCID}_{50} \text{ per mL} = 5 \times 10^{4.39}$$

References

1. Leigh R, Proud D (2015) Virus-induced modulation of lower airway diseases: pathogenesis and pharmacologic approaches to treatment. Pharmacol Ther 145:185–198
2. Arruda E, Boyle TR, Winther B, Pevear DC, Gwaltney JM Jr, Hayden FG (1995) Localization of human rhinovirus replication in the upper respiratory tract by in situ hybridization. J Infect Dis 171:1329–1333
3. Mosser AG, Brockman-Schneider R, Amineva S, Burchell L, Sedgewick JB, Busse WW, Gern JE (2002) Similar frequency of rhinovirus infectable cells in upper and lower airway epithelium. J Infect Dis 185:734–743
4. Winther B (2011) Rhinovirus infections in the upper airway. Proc Am Thorac Soc 8:79 89
5. Subauste MC, Jacoby DB, Richards SM, Proud D (1995) Infection of a human respiratory epithelial cell line with rhinovirus. Induction of cytokine release and modulation of susceptibility to infection by cytokine exposure. J Clin Invest 96:549–557
6. Winther B, Brofeldt S, Christensen B, Mygind N (1984) Light and scanning electron microscopy of nasal biopsy material from patients with naturally acquired common colds. Acta Otolarngol (Stockholm) 97:309–318
7. Reed LJ, Muench H (1938) A simple method of estimating fifty per cent endpoints. Amer J Hyg 27:493–497

Chapter 8

Analysis of Adherence Junctions in Rhinovirus-Infected Airway Epithelial Cells

Kevin Looi, Liisa M. Hirvonen, and Anthony Kicic

Abstract

The airway mucosal epithelium is the main gateway of entry for numerous human respiratory viruses, including human influenza virus, respiratory syncytial virus (RSV), coronavirus, and rhinoviruses (RV). For respiratory viruses to perpetuate infection, they must be able to traverse the airway mucosal epithelium and then spread into distal sites of the respiratory tract and lung parenchyma. However, this cellular interface has evolved well-developed apical junctional complexes (AJCs), including tight and adherens junctions, that bridge adjacent epithelial cells together. The resulting structure not only provides a strong physical barrier but also plays an active role in preventing and/or limiting the spread and dissemination of viral pathogens. Respiratory viruses, such as RVs, have been shown to target various components of these AJCs, either directly or indirectly, thus facilitating paracellular viral penetration, resulting in airway epithelial barrier dysfunction. Disruption of these AJCs may also result in unintended contact with hidden viral receptors, further enabling viral infection of the airway epithelium. Here we describe the various models of RV-infected airway epithelial cells and the methods used for the characterization and analysis of AJCs following RV infection.

Key words Tight junctions, Adherens junctions, Apical junctional complex, Viral infection, Rhinovirus, Barrier disruption, Epithelial barrier, Confocal microscopy, Transepithelial electrical resistance, Epithelial permeability, In-Cell Western™, Super-resolution microscopy

1 Introduction

The respiratory airways are constantly in direct contact with the external environment and are thus an integral part of the innate immune system. They also play a critical role in maintaining airway homeostasis, in addition to their primary function of providing a physical barrier against exogenous airborne insults and pathogens. This barrier is achieved via a network of airway surface liquids, mucus, and airway epithelial cells, with its apical junctional complexes (AJCs) consisting of tight junctions (TJs) and adherens junctions (AJs). Together with other junctional complexes like Gap junctions, desmosomes, and hemidesmosomes, AJCs are

Umadevi Sajjan (ed.), *Rhinovirus: Methods and Protocols*, Methods in Molecular Biology, vol. 2903,
https://doi.org/10.1007/978-1-0716-4410-2_8,

responsible for (i) the maintenance of cellular polarity and attachment between neighboring cells and (ii) regulating the flux of ions, particles, and pathogens across the paracellular space via a gate-like process. Perturbations to this epithelial gating process can often occur either via mechanical or biological insults, such as bacterial or viral infections. Viruses are obligate parasites and need to hijack the host cellular machinery for replication and survival. To do so, viruses gain entry into the cells either via binding of the virus to specific AJC targets to initiate AJC protein internalization or via AJC protein disassembly by regulating the expression and/or localization of the protein. This then allows the virus unencumbered access into the sub-epithelial space (Fig. 1), binding to basolateral receptors which are ordinarily inaccessible due to the functioning epithelial barrier.

Viral-induced epithelial permeability can also result in the sub-epithelial invasion by allergens or bacterial pathogens, with consequent ramifications on worsening pulmonary health. Evidence has shown that RVs, colloquially known as the common cold virus, are responsible for almost one-half of the respiratory virus infections globally [1, 2] and are often transmitted via direct contact or through small aerosol droplets. It is also the leading cause of upper respiratory tract infections [3], often leading to considerable economic burdens in terms of medical visits and absenteeism from either school or work. Although once thought to cause benign airway illness, RV infections have now been associated with exacerbations in many acute and chronic lung diseases [4, 5] and over all ages. Previous studies have demonstrated that RV infection of either primary airway epithelial cells (AECs) or immortalized cell lines has been associated with decreased transepithelial electrical resistance (TEER) and a consequent increase in epithelial paracellular permeability. These studies also demonstrated alterations in AJCs following RV infection [6–8] and showed an overall decrease in claudin-1, −4, occludin, zonula occluden (ZO)-1, E-cadherin, and Crumbs3 protein expression, thus increasing epithelial paracellular permeability and allowing viral entry into the sub-epithelial space. It is important for us to understand the process by which epithelial barrier disruption occurs, as this is critical in determining future therapeutic targets. Furthermore, understanding the interaction between RV infection and the airway epithelial barrier is of immense significance, as this would provide us with a pathway toward identifying the mechanisms of RV-induced epithelial pathology and eventually aid in the comprehension of the role of the airway epithelial barrier in the fight against respiratory viral infections. Here, we describe the materials and methods used for assessing and analyzing junctional complexes in airway epithelial cells following RV infection in primary airway epithelial cells.

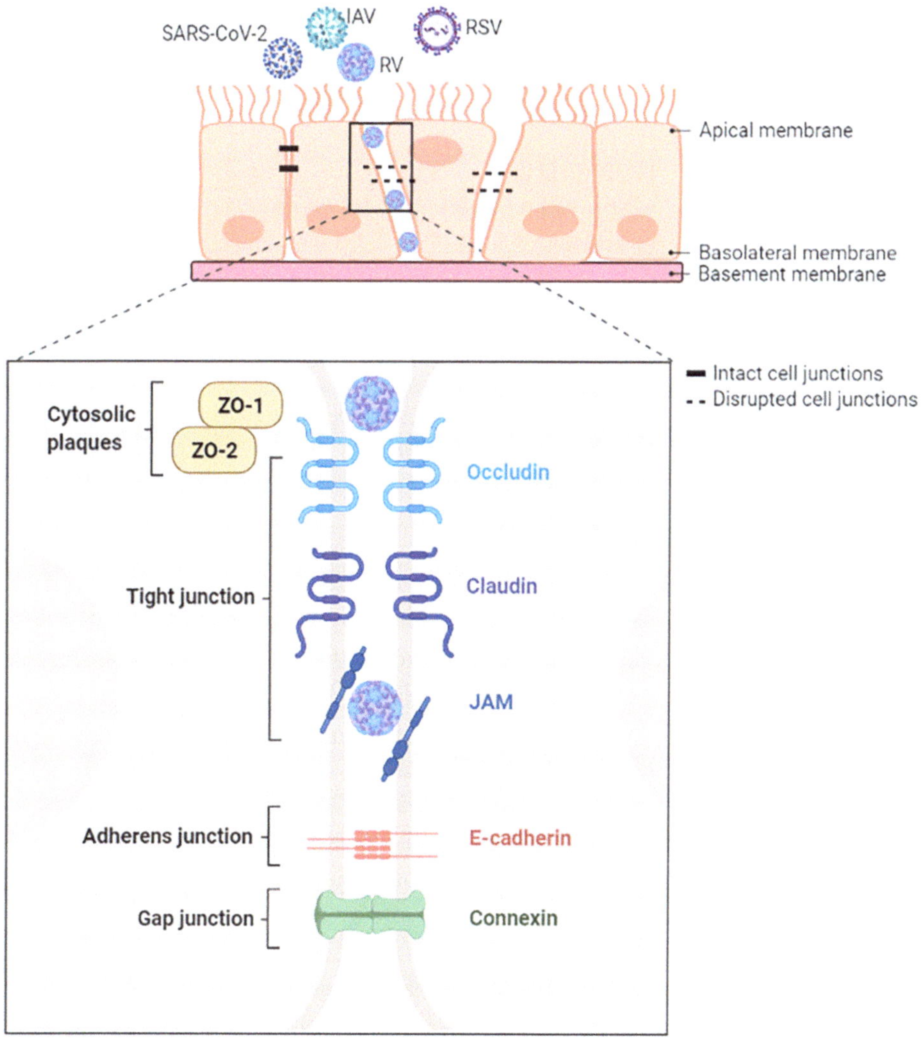

Fig. 1 Schematic of respiratory epithelial cell apical junction complex dissociating following RV infection. The airway mucosal epithelium consists of the airway surface liquids, mucus, and airway epithelial cells. Airway junctional complexes (AJCs) form between adjacent cells and comprise TJs, AJs, Gap junctions, and the cytosolic plaque proteins of the zonula occludens (ZO) family. Together with desmosomes and hemidesmosomes, they anchor the cells to the basement membrane. Respiratory viruses such as influenza (IAV), respiratory syncytial virus (RSV), rhinovirus (RV), and coronaviruses (SARS-CoV-2) can lead to AJC dissociation and disruption. Consequently, viral-induced epithelial permeability can result in further viral penetration, coming into contact with basolateral receptors that are ordinarily inaccessible. (Created with Biorender)

2 Materials

2.1 In-Cell™ Western Assay

1. Fixing Solution (3.7% (v/v) Formaldehyde): To 45-mL of 1 × PBS, add 5-mL of 37% Formaldehyde (Sigma-Aldrich, Catalog # 8.18708). Invert to mix and store away from direct light.

2. Triton Wash Solution: To 499.5-mL of 1 × PBS, add 0.5-mL of Triton ×-100 (Sigma-Aldrich, Catalog # ×100).
3. Tween Washing Solution: To 999-mL of 1 × PBS, add 1-mL of Tween-20 (Sigma-Aldrich, Catalog # P1379).

2.2 Transepithelial Permeability Assay

1. HEPES-HBSS: Dissolve 0.14-g/l $CaCl_2$, 0.1-g/l $MgCl_2 \bullet 6H_2O$, 0.1-g/l$MgSO_4 \bullet 7H_2O$, 0.4-g/l KCl, 0.06-g/l KH_2PO_4, 8.0-g/l NaCl, 0.04-g/l Na_2HPO_4, 1.0-g/l D-Glucose, 5.96-g/l HEPES, 0.35-g/l $NaHCO_3$ in 1000-mL of double distilled H_2O. Adjust pH to 7.4 with NaOH and sterilize with 0.22-μM bottle-top filter and store at room temperature.
2. FITC-dextran (4 or 20kDA; Sigma-Aldrich Catalog # FD-4, FD-20): Dissolve 20-mg of FITC-dextran in 10-mL of HEPES-HBSS. Sub-aliquot into 1.5-mL microtube and store at −20 °C.

2.3 Immunofluorescence

1. Acetone (Sigma-Aldrich, Catalog # 179124) and methanol (Sigma-Aldrich, Catalog # 34860) for fixation.
2. Permeabilization buffer: 0.1% (v/v) Saponin (Sigma-Aldrich, Catalog # S7900) in 1 × TBS.
3. Blocking buffer: 10% (v/v) normal goat serum (Sigma-Aldrich, Catalog # G9023), 10% (v/v) fetal bovine serum (Sigma-Aldrich, Catalog # 12003C) and 1% (v/v) bovine serum albumin (Sigma-Aldrich, Catalog # A7030) in 1 × TBS.
4. Mouse or rabbit anti-apical junctional complex primary antibodies.
5. Secondary antibodies (Anti-mouse or Anti-rabbit) with fluorescent labels: (ThermoFisher, AF-488, Catalog # A-11001, A-11008; AF-568, Catalog # A-11004, A-11011), anti-mouse iFluor-647 (AAT Bioquest, Catalog # 16783), anti-rabbit iFluor-647 (AAT Bioquest, Catalog # 16837).
6. DAPI (ThermoFisher, 4′,6-Diamidino-2-Phenylindole, Dihydrochloride, Catalog # D1306).

2.4 Microscopy

1. ProLong™ Diamond Antifade Mount (ThermoFisher, Catalog # P36961).
2. For confocal and SIM microscopy: microscope slides and #1.5 coverslips (high-precision 170 μm coverslips for SIM), nail polish containing non-fluorescent pigments.
3. For STORM: 35 mm dishes with #1.5 coverslip bottoms; e.g., P35G-1.5-10-C (MatTek), FD35 (WPI), or μ-Dish (ibidi).
4. STORM buffer: TN buffer: H_2O with 50 mM Tris pH 8.0 and 10 mM NaCl. MEA stock solution: 1 M cysteamine (Sigma–Aldrich, Catalog # 30070) in H_2O, pH adjusted to 8.0 with

HCl solution. Prepare STORM buffer by adding MEA stock to TN buffer at a final concentration of 50 mM immediately before imaging (*see* **Note 1**).

5. Confocal microscopy: A confocal microscope with 3 channels (405 nm excitation for Hoechst 33342, 488 nm excitation for AF-488, and 561 nm excitation for AF-568), and high NA oil immersion objective lens with at least 40× magnification (*see* **Note 2**).
6. SIM microscopy: A structured illumination microscope with channels matching fluorescent labels (e.g., 405, 488 and 568 nm excitation), a 3D imaging option, and image reconstruction software (*see* **Note 3**).
7. STORM microscopy: A microscope with SMLM image capture option on the 647 nm channel (i.e., with a 640–647 nm laser, wide-field illumination, and a fast camera) and SMLM image reconstruction software (*see* **Note 4**).

3 Methods

3.1 Assessing AJC Gene Expression from Primary AECs

3.1.1 Extraction

1. Repetitive pipetting up and down to ensure complete lysis of cells by Qiazol/Trizol. Incubate the lysate at room temperature for an additional 5 min to allow complete dissociation of nucleoprotein complexes.
2. Add 0.2-mL chloroform per 1-mL Qiazol/Trizol Reagent used. Shake vigorously by hand for 15 s. Incubate at room temperature for 3 min.
3. That is, 70-μL of chloroform for 350-μL Qiazol/Trizol reagent used.
4. Centrifuge sample at 12,000 *g* for 15 min at 4 °C (*see* **Note 5**).
5. Transfer the upper aqueous phase containing the RNA to a fresh RNase-free tube.
6. Add 1 volume of 70% (v/v) ethanol to obtain a final ethanol concentration of 35%. Vortex to mix well (*see* **Note 6**).
7. Invert the tube to disperse any visible precipitate that may form after adding ethanol.
8. Transfer the sample (<700-μL) to a spin cartridge, centrifuge at 12,000 *g* for 15 s at room temperature. Discard flow through (*see* **Note 7**).
9. Add 350-μL Wash Buffer I to spin cartridge, centrifuge at 12,000 *g* for 15 s at room temperature. Discard the flow-through.

10. Performed on column PureLink DNase treatment. Add 80-μL of the following mixture into each spin cartridge membrane and incubate for 15 min.

Component	Volume (μL)
10× DNase I reaction buffer	8
Resuspended DNase (~3 U/μL)	10
RNase-free water	62

11. Repeat **step 8**. Transfer the spin cartridge to a new collection tube.
12. Add 500 μL of Wash Buffer II onto the column and centrifuge at 12,000 *g* for 15 s at room temperature. Discard the flow-through.
13. Repeat **step 11**.
14. Centrifuge at 12,000 *g* for 1 min at room temperature to dry the membrane. Discard the collection tube and transfer the spin cartridge into a recovery tube.
15. Add 30–100-μL RNase–free water to elute RNA, incubate at RT for 1 min, and centrifuge at 12,000 *g* for 2 min at room temperature.
16. Assess isolated RNA for quality and quantity by measuring spectrophotometric absorbance at 260 and 280 nm using a NanoDrop.

3.1.2 RT-PCR

1. Prepare master mix according to the number of samples or reactions (usually prepare N + 1).
2. Master Mix preparation. Work out the amount of RNA for each reaction (preferably 200 ng) and water to make up to 20 μL/reaction.

Master mix	1 reaction (μL)	Final concentration
10× RT buffer	2	1×
25 mM $MgCl_2$	4.4	5.5 mM
40 mM dNTP mix	1	2 mM mix (0.5 mM each dNTP)
Random hexamers	1	2.5 μM
Rnase inhibitor	0.4	8 units
MultiScribe reverse transcriptase	0.5	25 units
RNA (200 ng) and H_2O	X	
Total volume	20	

3. Run samples using a thermal cycler on a standard reverse transcription program at 25 °C for 10 min, 48 °C for 60 min, 95 °C for 5 min, and lastly, 4 °C for infinity.

3.1.3 Quantitative PCR

1. Make up master mix for each of the apical junctional complex genes of interest and housekeeping gene of your selection, with approximately 10% more of the total number of samples. Total volume per reaction is 20 μL.

Master mix	1 reaction (μL)
2× TaqMan master mix	10
Primer/probe mix	1
H_2O	4
cDNA	5

2. Pipette master mix into each well. Once done, put caps on each "column" of the plate (if using a 96-well plate) or on each "strip" if using a strip of 8 tubes.
3. Take off caps per column or remove the PCR plate sealer when ready to dispense cDNA samples into each well. Once finished with that column, put the caps back on to avoid contamination.
4. Once all samples are done, push caps tightly or reseal with a plate sealer.
5. Short vortex to mix samples and spin down.
6. Run samples using the Applied Biosystem QuantStudio7 on a standard QuantStudio7 Flex system TaqMan program.

3.2 Assessing AJC Protein Expression from Primary AECs

In-Cell™ Western Assay.

Day 1:

1. Remove cell culture media. Immediately fix cells with 150 μL of fresh fixing solution for 20 min at room temperature without shaking. If cell permeabilization is not required, proceed to **step 3** (*see* **Note 8**).
2. To permeabilize, wash with 200 μL of Triton Wash Solution in each well for 5 min per wash on an orbital shaker. Remove wash manually and do not allow cells/wells to become dry during washing. Repeat the wash process for a total of 5 washes.
3. Add 150 μL of fresh Odyssey Blocking Buffer to each well and allow blocking for 1.5 h at room temperature with moderate shaking on an orbital shaker.
4. Dilute desired primary antibodies in fresh blocking buffer or another appropriate blocker of choice. As a general

guideline, 1:50 to 1:200 dilutions are recommended depending on the primary antibody. If the antibody supplier provides dilution guidelines for western blot staining, start with that recommended range and determine empirically.

5. Remove the blocking buffer from **step 3** and store it in 50-mL tubes. Blocking buffer can be reused for up to 3 times.
6. Add 50 μL of fresh blocking buffer to the control wells and 50 μL of the desired primary antibody diluted in blocking buffer to the remaining wells.
7. Incubate with primary antibody for 2.5 h at room temperature with moderate shaking on an orbital shaker **OR** overnight at 4 °C with gentle shaking.

   Day 1 (Cont'd)/Day 2 (Overnight incubation):

8. Remove primary antibody dilutions and wash with 200 μL of Tween Wash Solution in each well for 5 min per wash on an orbital shaker. Remove wash manually and do not allow cells/wells to become dry during washing. Repeat the wash process for a total of 5 washes.
9. Dilute fluorescently labelled secondary antibodies in fresh blocking buffer. The recommended dilution range is 1:200 to 1:1200, with a suggested starting dilution of 1:800. The optimal dilution required should be determined empirically.

Secondary antibody mix (complete)	
Fluorescently labelled secondary antibody	Dilution to be determined by user
DRAQ5™	1:10000
Sapphire700™	1:1000
Tween-20	0.2% (final concentration)
Block buffer	Top up to required total volume

10. Add 50 μL of secondary antibody mix ***without*** DRAQ5 and Sapphire700 to the control wells and 50 μL of secondary antibody mix (complete) to the rest of the wells.
11. Incubate for 1 h at room temperature with gentle shaking. Protect the plate from light during incubation.
12. Remove the secondary antibody mix and wash with 200 μL of Tween Wash Solution in each well for 5 min per wash on an orbital shaker. Remove wash manually and do not allow cells/wells to become dry during washing. Repeat the

wash process for a total of 5 washes. Protect the plate from light during washing.

13. After the final wash, remove the wash solution completely and gently tap/blot the plate on laboratory bench wipes to remove traces of Tween Wash Solution. For best results, scan plate *immediately*; plates may be stored at 4 °C for up to 2 weeks (protected from ambient light).
14. Before scanning the plate, clean the bottom plate surface and Odyssey CLx Imager scanning bed with moist, lint-free paper.
15. Scan plate with detection in both 700 and 800 channels. Generally, a scan resolution of 169 μm is appropriate. Initial intensity setting of 5 is suggested for both channels but should be determined empirically by the User. A focus offset of 3 is suggested but should also be determined by User (*see* Fig. 2a–c).
16. Proceed with data analysis using Image Studio software (Fig. 2d, e).

3.3 Assessing Barrier Function and Integrity in Well-Differentiated Primary AECs

3.3.1 Transepithelial Electrical Resistance (TEER) Measurement

1. Disinfect the STX2 "chopsticks" electrode (World Precision Instruments, USA) in 80% (v/v) ethanol and place it in fresh HEPES-HBSS for a few minutes.
2. Connect the electrode to the EVOM^2 volt-ohm meter (World Precision Instruments, USA) by inserting the RJ plug at the end of the flexible electrode cable into the input port of the meter. Turn the meter on and allow a few minutes for equilibration.
3. Remove the cell culture media and replace it with fresh HEPES-HBSS for both the culture scaffold (200 μL) and culture well (1 mL).
4. Measure the resistance of a blank (i.e., cell culture scaffold without cells) filled with HEPES-HBSS by inserting the electrode with the shorter arm into the culture scaffold and the longer arm touching the bottom of the culture well. Allow for a steady ohms reading of the solution resistance (*see* **Note 9**).
5. Perform the experimental resistance measurements in triplicate readings. To obtain the true resistance value, average the triplicate readings and subtract the blank resistance. From there, to obtain the unit area resistance, multiply the true resistance value by the effective surface area of the culture insert membrane (*see* **Note 10**).

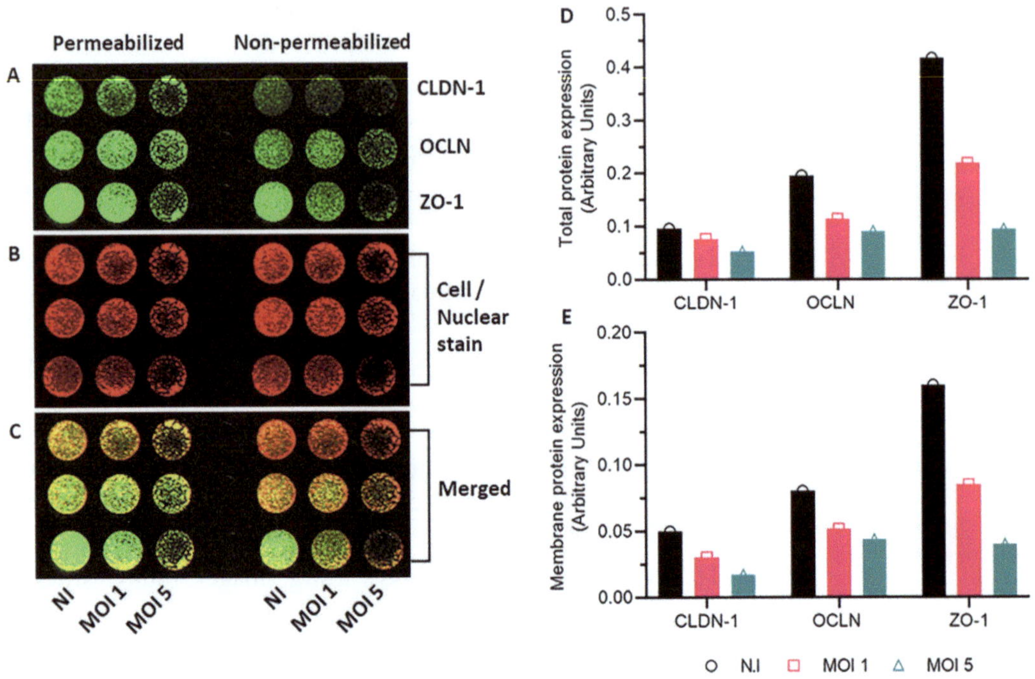

Fig. 2 Effect of RV infection on primary AECs TJ signal intensity and expression. Primary AECs derived from children without asthma and atopy, seeded onto 96-well black microplates and grown to confluence, were infected with 2 different multiplicities of infection (MOI) of RV. Incubation with primary antibodies to claudin (CLDN)-1, occludin (OCLN), and zonula occluden (ZO)-1 was performed overnight, followed by incubation with IRDye™ secondary antibodies. (**a**) Permeabilized (Total) and non-permeabilized (Membrane) TJ signal intensity observed at the 800 nm channel showed the effect of RV infection after 24 h infection. (**b**) Uniform cell densities in all wells following staining with Sapphire700™ and Draq5™ indicate a confluent monolayer as observed at the 700 nm channel. (**c**) Merged image of (**a**) and (**b**) is used for the quantification of TJ protein expression as normalized to cell densities. (**d** and **e**) Representative graphs of total and membrane signal intensities of CLDN-1, OCLN, and ZO-1 in primary AEC monolayer following RV infection post normalization to cell densities. Highest signal intensities were observed in non-infected (NI) cells, followed by cells infected with MOI 1 and MOI 5 of RV, respectively

3.3.2 Transepithelial Permeability Assay

1. Collect cell culture media, transfer it to 1.5-mL microtube, and immediately place it on ice.
2. Add 0.2 mL of HEPES-HBSS to insert and 1 mL to cell culture well. Return to incubator for 15 min at 37 °C.
3. While waiting for **step 2**, transfer:
   (a) 0.05 mL of FITC-Dextran 4 and/or 20 kDa solution to "Timepoint 0-AP" 0.5-mL microtube.
   (b) 0.05 mL of HEPES-buffered HBSS to separate "Timepoint 0-BL" 0.5-mL microtube.
4. Measure TEER prior to the start of the permeability assay.
5. Collect apical wash from insert (0.2 mL) into a 0.5-mL microtube and immediately place it on ice.

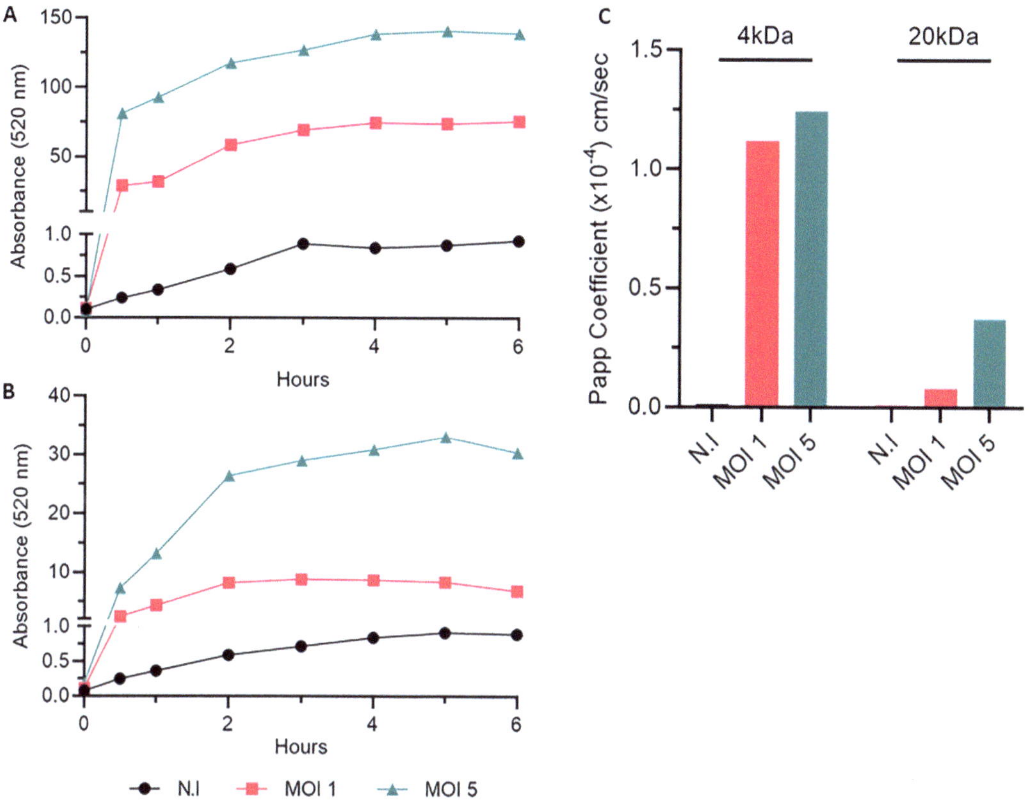

Fig. 3 Effect of RV infection on epithelial permeability of FITC-dextran molecules across well-differentiated multilayered primary AECs. Cells were cultured on Corning transwell inserts, grown to confluence, and allowed to polarize and differentiate for up to 28 days. Infection with multiplicities of infection (MOI) 1 and MOI 5 of RV was performed, and a transepithelial permeability assay was conducted to assess the throughput of both 4 kDa and 20 kDa FITC-dextran molecules. (**a**) Representative graphs of a minor increase in 4 kDa FITC-dextran molecule concentration in the basolateral compartment is observed up to 6 h for non-infected (N.I) cells. Larger increase in the basolateral compartment concentration was observed for cells infected with MOI 1, with the greatest increase in concentration observed in cells infected with MOI 5, over a 6 h sampling time. (**b**) Representative graphs of a minor increase in 20 kDa FITC-dextran molecule concentration in the basolateral compartment is observed up to 6 h for non-infected (N.I) cells. Larger increase in basolateral compartment concentration was observed for cells infected with MOI 1, with the greatest increase in concentration observed in cells infected with MOI 5, over a 6 h sampling time. (**c**) Representative graphical summary of the apparent permeability (P_{app}) of 4 and 20 kDa FITC-dextran molecule in N.I cells and cultures infected with MOI 1 and MOI 5

6. Aspirate HEPES-HBSS from culture wells and replace it with 1-mL fresh HEPES-HBSS in wells.
7. To inserts, add 0.2 mL of FITC-Dextran 4 **OR** 20 kDa solution apically.
8. Incubate the culture inserts on an orbital shaker at 37 °C to minimize unstirred water level.

9. Sample 0.5 mL from the basolateral culture well and replace it with fresh 0.5 mL of HEPES-HBSS at pre-determined time points (i.e., 0.5, 1, 2, 3, 4, 5, and 6 h).
10. At each timepoint, transfer the 0.5-mL collected HEPES-HBSS into a pre-labelled 0.5-mL microtube and store it in the fridge, away from direct light.
11. For the final time point (i.e., 6 h), collect apical FITC-dextran solution from inserts and 0.5 mL from wells and transfer to 0.5-mL microtube.
12. Aspirate all remaining HEPES-HBSS from basolateral culture wells.
13. Add 0.2 mL (inserts) and 1 mL (culture wells) of fresh HEPES-HBSS for the final wash.
14. Place back into incubator for 15 min.
15. Remove all remaining HEPES-HBSS and proceed to fix for confocal laser scanning or super-resolution microscopy (*see* **Note 11**).
16. From the 0.5-mL HEPES-HBSS collected at each timepoint, transfer 0.05 mL into a 96-well black microplate (Greinerbio, Catalog # 655077) and read using a multi-label plate reader (excitation 492 nm/emission 520 nm).
17. Apparent permeability (P_{app}) of FITC-dextran from the apical to the basolateral compartment is calculated following the general equation: $P_{app} = (dQ/dt) \times (1/AC_0)$, where dQ/dt is the steady-state flux, A is the surface area of the membrane, and C_0 is the initial concentration in the apical compartment (Fig. 3).

3.4 AJC Visualization

3.4.1 Sample Preparation for Microscopy

1. Fix the samples with appropriate fixative [9], followed by washing with 1 × TBS for 30 min at room temperature, replacing wash TBS every 5 min (*see* **Note 12**).
2. Permeabilize by incubating in permeabilization buffer for 10 min at room temperature. Wash with 1 × TBS for 30 min at room temperature, replacing wash TBS every 5 min.
3. To minimize non-specific binding of primary and secondary antibodies in samples, incubate in blocking buffer for 30 min at room temperature.
4. Dilute appropriate primary antibody in blocking buffer. If the antibody supplier provides dilution guidelines for immunofluorescent staining, start with that recommended range. The optimal dilution required should be determined empirically. Incubate samples for 1 h at room temperature, followed by washing with 1 × TBS at room temperature every 10 min for 1 h.

5. For confocal laser scanning microscopy and SIM, dilute the appropriate secondary antibody, as determined empirically, in blocking buffer. For STORM imaging, use an iFluor-647 secondary antibody at a 1 mg/mL concentration. Protect the samples from light and incubate for 1 h at room temperature, followed by washing with 1 × TBS at room temperature every 10 min for 1 h. During the final wash step, add DAPI to counterstain for nuclei.
6. Store in 1 × TBS at 4 °C until needed for imaging.

3.4.2 Confocal Laser Scanning Microscopy

1. Mount samples on slides with mounting medium, place a #1.5 coverslip on top, and seal the coverslip onto the slide with nail polish. Protect the samples from light and leave to dry thoroughly.
2. Place the sample in the confocal microscope. If high-resolution imaging is required, determine the appropriate image resolution required to achieve Nyquist sampling for the chosen objective lens.
3. Set the pinhole to 1.2 airy units. To minimize bleed-through, set the microscope to capture individual channels sequentially rather than simultaneously. Focus on to the brightest plane.
4. Optimize the laser power and gain settings for each individual channel (*see* **Note 13**). Select one fluorescence channel and switch off the others. Using a look-up table (LUT) to observe the pixel intensity histogram, adjust the laser power simultaneously with the detector gain until the pixels with the highest intensities are just slightly below the value required to oversaturate the signal. Keep the sample exposure to a minimum to prevent photobleaching of the sample (*see* **Note 14**).
5. Once optimized, switch off this channel and repeat the optimization for other channels (Fig. 4a–f).
6. Determine the optimum spacing (step size) for a Z-stack. This depends on the objective but is typically around 0.2–0.5 μm for high-resolution imaging. Focus the sample up and down and set the Z-range by visually determining the top and bottom of the sample.
7. Acquire a Z-stack. Record and document all settings identified during microscope setup and configuration. These will be used for repeating the experiment for samples cultured under the different conditions (e.g., infected with a virus) (Fig. 4d–f).

3.4.3 Structured Illumination Microscopy (SIM)

While confocal microscopy is a standard imaging method in biology, its resolution is limited to about half the wavelength of the light, or about ~200–240 nm, by diffraction. SIM is a "super-resolution" technique that uses mathematical image reconstruction

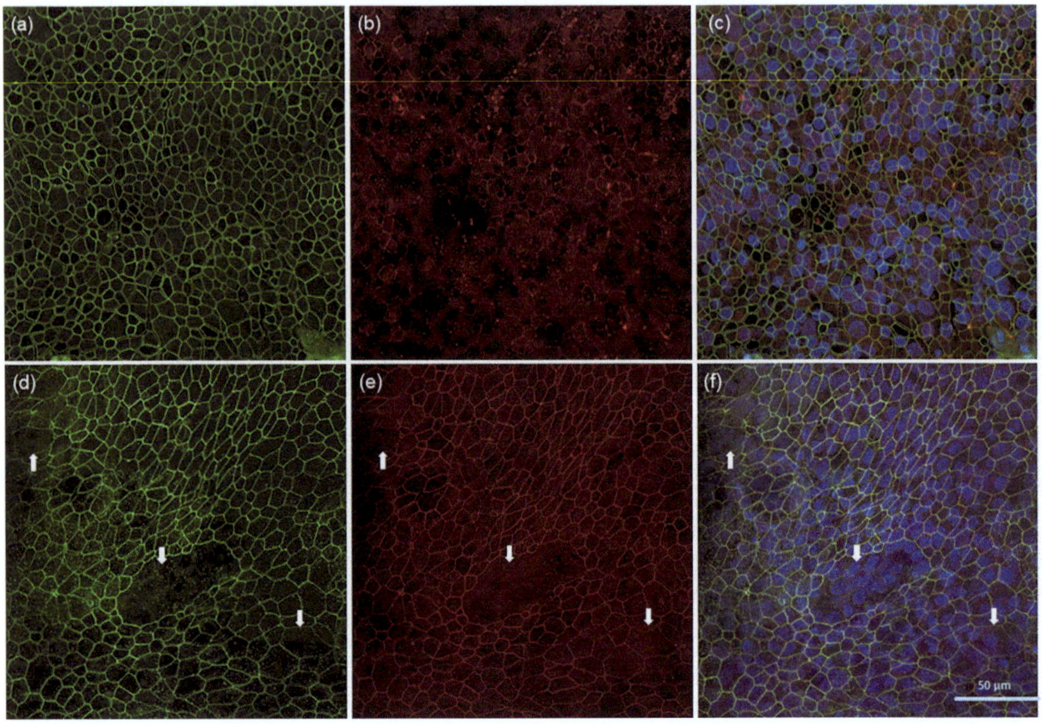

Fig. 4 Visualization of membrane TJ protein expression in well-differentiated, multilayered cultures derived from primary AECs of children without asthma and atopy following RV infection with confocal laser scanning microscopy. Culture scaffolds with primary AECs were fixed and incubated with primary antibodies to ZO-1 (Green; **a** and **d**) and occludin (OCLN) (Red; **b** and **e**) for 1 h at room temperature, followed by secondary antibodies for 1 h in the dark at room temperature. Cultures were then counterstained with DAPI, which illuminates cellular nuclear material (Blue). (**a–c**) Confocal imaging of ZO-1 and OCLN in representative samples from non-infected primary AECs demonstrates an even, uninterrupted cobblestone appearance of both TJs. (**d–f**) Confocal imaging of ZO-1 and OCLN in representative samples from primary AECs infected with MOI 1 of RV demonstrates areas of TJ disruption and loss in expression (white arrows). (Images are representative of $n = 6$ (Total magnification 60× Oil)

to improve resolution beyond this diffraction limit [10]. Resolution improvement by SIM is limited to a maximum of a factor of two compared to conventional light microscopy, leading to a typical resolution of ~120 nm. SIM can be operated in either 2D or 3D mode. 2D mode requires fewer raw images and is therefore faster but is more suited for flat samples, e.g., cells grown on coverslips. For imaging junctional complexes in well-differentiated, multilayered samples that are typically not flat, 3D imaging is able to give a more complete picture of junctions that are not on one plane, as well as providing the benefit of optical sectioning and reduced out-of-focus blur (Fig. 5a–d).

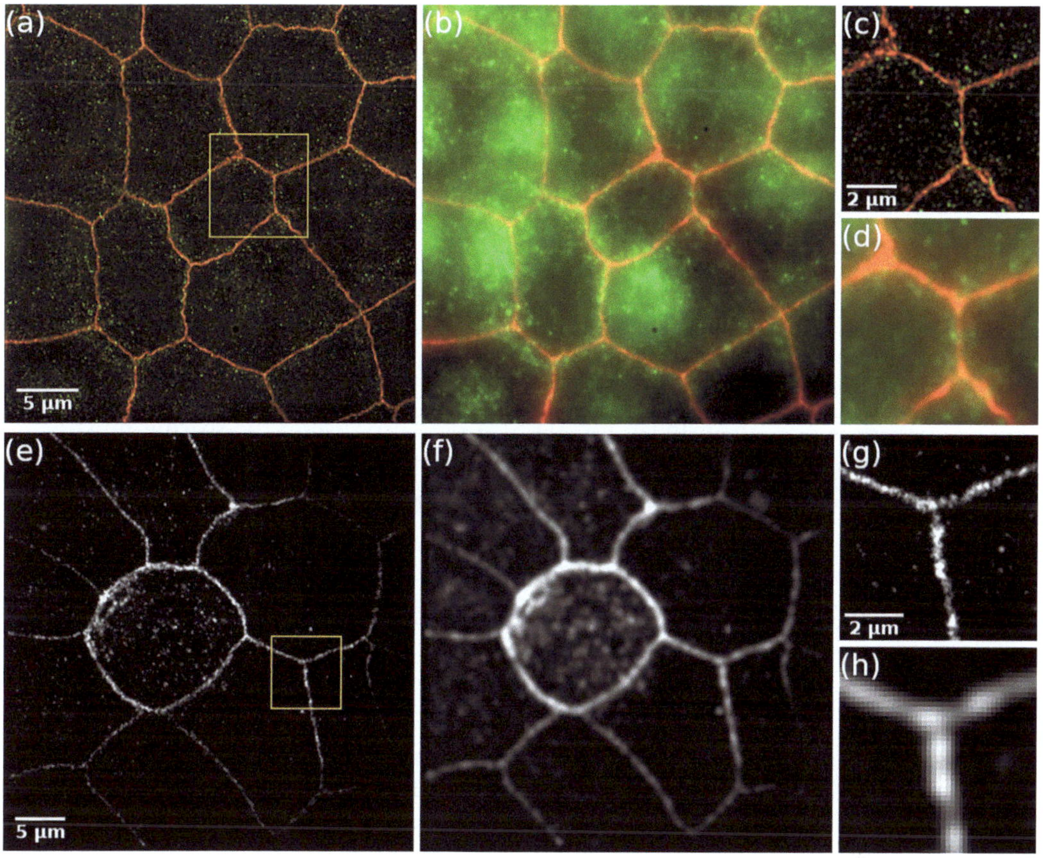

Fig. 5 Visualization of membrane TJ protein expression in well-differentiated, multilayered cultures derived from primary AECs of children without asthma and atopy with super-resolution microscopy. Culture scaffolds with primary AECs were fixed and incubated with primary antibody to zonula occluden (ZO)-1 (Red, **a**–**d**) for 1 h at room temperature, followed by secondary antibodies for 1 h in the dark at room temperature. (**a**, **c**) SIM imaging can enhance resolution by a factor of two, to about 100 nm, compared to (**b**, **d**) conventional wide-field microscopy. STORM can improve this further, typically to ~30–50 nm; STORM imaging (**e**, **g**) of iFluor-647-labelled ZO-1 shows clear resolution improvement compared to wide-field imaging (**f**, **h**) of the same area. Right column (**c**, **d**, **g**, **h**) shows enlarged areas indicated with orange rectangles in (**a**, **e**)

1. Mount samples on slides with mounting medium, place a #1.5 high-precision coverslip on top, and seal the coverslip onto the slide with nail polish. Protect the samples from light and leave to dry thoroughly.
2. Select a high-magnification oil immersion objective (e.g., 100×) to match the refractive index (RI) of the mounting medium. Using the eyepiece, bring the sample to rough focus.
3. Switch to digital imaging and select a channel that shows the labelled junctions. Using low laser power, bring the sample to the best focus, and select an area for imaging. Try to select a flat area, as a large focus range will lead to long image acquisition times.

4. Select the imaging mode that will be used for SIM imaging (e.g., 3D SIM). Optimize the laser power, camera exposure time, and camera gain such that the image brightness is within the optimum range (camera linear range, as specified in your SIM manual), and laser power is low enough to not photobleach the sample.
5. Once optimized, repeat this process for other color channels.
6. Set Z-stack parameters. Select a channel that shows the labelled junctions. Focus the sample up and down and set the Z-range top and bottom by visually determining the top and bottom of the sample. Typically, a minimum of 7 slices are required for 3D reconstruction. Ensure that the Z-spacing is as specified in your manual; for 3D SIM data processing, the spacing must be as specified and cannot be changed.
7. Set the channel acquisition order. Select the channels that you have optimized for imaging, and ensure that they are in the order of importance (i.e., most important first), as some photobleaching may occur during imaging.
8. Run the 3D SIM acquisition. Once complete, check for data integrity; SIM processing will not work if there is sample drift or photobleaching that occurs during the stack acquisition.
9. Run the 3D SIM processing. If the results show clear artifacts, e.g., a grid pattern over the image, adjust the processing parameters until a better result is achieved. Note that artifacts arising from problems in the raw data, e.g., sample drift or photobleaching, cannot be corrected during processing. Poor signal-to-noise ratio will also lead to poor-quality reconstruction.
10. Create a maximum intensity projection of the result for a "2D" view and save all images.

3.4.4 STORM Imaging

Single-molecule localization microscopy (SMLM) is another super-resolution technique that can image beyond the diffraction limit. In SMLM the fluorescent labels are made to blink, and a series of images is acquired where only a few molecules are emitting in each frame. This allows the center position of each molecule to be determined with high accuracy, and the final high-resolution image is then obtained by summing thousands of frames together [11]. SMLM can provide theoretically unlimited resolution; in practice, this is limited by the signal-to-noise ratio, typically to about 20–50 nm. STochastic Optical Reconstruction Microscopy (STORM) is a SMLM technique that uses specific dyes and buffers to induce the blinking. This protocol uses the fluorescent dye iFluor-647 to label the junctions and a buffer containing a thiol to induce the blinking [12]; example images are shown in Fig. 5e–h.

1. Invert a sample labelled with the STORM dye iFluor-647 onto a 35-mm dish with a coverslip bottom.
2. Prepare 1 mL of STORM buffer by adding MEA stock to TN buffer at a final concentration of 50 mM. Aspirate any liquid from the dish and add the STORM buffer immediately before imaging. Once the buffer is added to the dish, imaging time is limited to a couple of hours.
3. Select the STORM objective; usually this is a high-magnification oil immersion objective (e.g., 100×). Using the eyepiece, bring the sample into a rough focus.
4. Switch to digital imaging and select the STORM channel. Ensure that the correct magnification and mode (2D) are selected for STORM imaging. Using low laser power (~0.5–1%) and exposure time of ~200–500 ms, bring the sample to the best focus (*see* **Note 15**).
5. Choose an area for imaging and adjust the image size by changing the number of pixels (*see* **Note 16**).
6. Adjust the angle for total internal reflection (TIRF) away from complete TIRF and towards oblique illumination until the required imaging depth is achieved (*see* **Note 17**).
7. Set the STORM parameters: number of frames (typically 10,000–20,000), exposure time (typically 10–30 ms), and laser power (depends on the laser and the illumination area, typically 30–100%) (*see* **Note 18**).
8. Start STORM acquisition. Monitor the acquisition and increase laser power during acquisition if required to sustain blinking. If the sample bleaches and the blinking stops, finish the acquisition.
9. Once the acquisition is completed, process the data according to the STORM manual using the vendor's software. This will give you a good indication of the quality of the data.
10. For more advanced processing, there are many SMLM data processing programs that can provide additional resources. A Fiji plugin, ThunderSTORM [13], allows flexible reconstruction of many types of STORM data. Pre-processing methods such as HAWK [14] can be used to separate overlapping molecules, which reduces artifacts in the final image and shortens data collection time by enabling higher density data processing.

4 Notes

1. MEA stock solution can be stored at 4 °C for up to 4 weeks.
2. We utilize a Nikon A1 inverted microscope (Nikon, Japan), with a Nikon Plan Apo VC 60× NA 1.4 oil immersion

objective (Nikon, Japan) and NIS-AR Elements software (Nikon, Japan).

3. We use a Nikon SIM (Ti2) microscope with a Nikon SR Apo TIRF 100×/1.49 NA oil immersion objective, 405, 488, and 561 nm excitation laser, an Andor iXon 897 EMCCD camera for image capture, and Nikon NIS Elements software for image reconstruction.
4. We use a Nikon STORM (Ti-E) microscope with a Nikon HP Apo TIRF 100×/1.49NA oil immersion objective, a 647 nm excitation laser, and a Hamamatsu OCRA FLASH 4 sCMOS camera for image capture. The raw data was pre-processed with HAWK software [13], and the super-resolution images were reconstructed with the Fiji plugin ThunderSTORM [12].
5. After centrifugation, the mixture separates into a lower red phenol-chloroform phase, an interphase, and a colorless upper aqueous phase which contains the RNA.
6. Ethanol used for RNA extraction should always be molecular biology-grade pure ethanol.
7. If sample volumes are greater than 700 μL, repeat the step until the entire sample is processed.
8. Primary AECs are seeded on a 96-well black microplate (Greinerbio, Catalog # 655077) at a density of 8.5×10^4 cells/cm^2, and culture media is refreshed every alternate day until a confluent cell monolayer is achieved. Triplicate wells are generally set up for each condition and each AJC to be assessed. RV infection is then performed, with the calculated titers and for the required length of infection (i.e., 6, 12, 24, 48, or 72 h).
9. The blank resistance must be measured and then subtracted from the final resistance reading across the culture inserts with cells to obtain the true resistance measurement.
10. The resistance is inversely proportional to the surface area. Thus, the larger the membrane, the lower the resistance. The unit of measurement is Ω.cm^2.
11. The choice of fixative is determined by whether the culture insert is subsequently used for routine histological stains and light microscopy or epifluorescence stains and high-resolution microscopy.
12. The type of fixative used to obtain optimal staining for claudin-1, occludin, and ZO-1 has been previously determined [9]. Fixative for other junctional complexes will need to be determined empirically.
13. The laser power needs to be set to the lowest possible value required to generate an image without photobleaching a sample.

14. Most confocal microscopy software includes a special Look Up Table (LUT) that will specifically indicate the presence of pixels that are over-saturated or under-saturated. If this is not possible, use the intensity histogram to ensure most of the dynamic range is covered without saturating any pixels.
15. STORM can also be performed in 3D mode, but here 2D imaging is sufficient since the aim of this experiment is not to measure distances in the axial direction. As a wide-field technique, STORM has a large depth of focus compared to confocal imaging.
16. Due to the large number of frames required for STORM image reconstruction, it is usually best to limit the imaging area to 256×256 pixels, or smaller if more than 20,000 frames are acquired.
17. SMLM is often performed in TIRF mode, which limits the illumination depth to ~100 nm. For well-differentiated, multilayered samples that are not flat, it is better to use oblique illumination with increased illumination depth.
18. Use a different area or a test sample to determine these parameters prior to imaging your sample. The laser power should be high enough such that the molecules blink fast, and the optimum exposure time depends on the blinking speed and density. With sustained blinking, a higher number of frames gives a better final image, but if the sample bleaches during the acquisition, then acquisition should be stopped to avoid unnecessary increases in noise and file size.

References

1. Lee W-M, Robert F, Lemanske J, Evans MD, Vang F, Pappas T, Gangnon R et al (2012) Human rhinovirus species and season of infection determine illness severity. Am J Respir Crit Care Med 186(9):886–891
2. Ng KT, Oong XY, Lim SH, Chook JB, Takebe Y, Chan YF et al (2018) Viral load and sequence analysis reveal the symptom severity, diversity, and transmission clusters of rhinovirus infections. Clin Infect Dis 67(2): 261–268
3. Kennedy JL, Turner RB, Braciale T, Heymann PW, Borish L (2012) Pathogenesis of rhinovirus infection. Curr Opin Virol 2(3):287–293
4. Bizzintino J, Lee W, Laing I, Vang F, Pappas T, Zhang G et al (2011) Association between human rhinovirus C and severity of acute asthma in children. Eur Respir J 37(5): 1037–1042
5. Mallia P, Kebadze T, Contoli M, Ward CK, Barnathan ES, Mascelli MA et al (2014) Airway inflammation and illness severity in response to experimental rhinovirus infection in asthma. Chest 145(6):1219–1229
6. Yeo N-K, Jang YJ (2010) Rhinovirus infection-induced alteration of tight junction and adherens junction components in human nasal epithelial cells. Laryngoscope 120(2):346–352
7. Sajjan U (2008) Rhinovirus disrupts the barrier function of polarized airway epithelial cells. Am J Respir Crit Care Med 178(12):1271
8. Looi K, Buckley A, Rigby P, Garratt L, Iosifidis T, Zosky G et al (2018) Effects of human rhinovirus on epithelial barrier integrity and function in children with asthma. Clin Exp Allergy 48(5):513–524
9. Buckley AG, Looi K, Iosifidis T, Ling K-M, Sutanto EN, Martinovich KM et al (2018) Visualisation of multiple tight junctional complexes in human airway epithelial cells. Biol Proc Online 20(1):3

10. Heintzmann R, Huser T (2017) Super-resolution structured illumination microscopy. Chem Rev 117(23):13890–13908
11. Lelek M, Gyparaki MT, Beliu G, Schueder F, Griffié J, Manley S et al (2021) Single-molecule localization microscopy. Nat Rev Methods Primers 1(1):1–27
12. Hirvonen LM, Cox S (2018) STORM without enzymatic oxygen scavenging for correlative atomic force and fluorescence superresolution microscopy. Methods Appl Fluores 6(4): 045002
13. Ovesný M, Křížek P, Borkovec J, Švindrych Z, Hagen GM (2014) ThunderSTORM: a comprehensive ImageJ plug-in for PALM and STORM data analysis and super-resolution imaging. Bioinformatics 30(16):2389–2390
14. Marsh RJ, Pfisterer K, Bennett P, Hirvonen LM, Gautel M, Jones GE et al (2018) Artifact-free high-density localization microscopy analysis. Nat Methods 15(9):689–692

Chapter 9

Culturing of Airway Stem Cells Obtained from COPD Patients to Assess the Effects of Rhinovirus Infection

Mohsen Tabasi, Tyler Markward, and Umadevi Sajjan

Abstract

Rhinovirus primarily infects airway epithelial cells lining the conductive airways. Mucociliary-differentiated airway epithelial cell cultures, established from airway basal cells, are relevant in vitro model systems to examine the rhinovirus-stimulated innate immune responses and changes in barrier function. The airway epithelium in patients with chronic respiratory diseases such as asthma, cystic fibrosis, and chronic obstructive pulmonary disease often shows remodeling, such as goblet cell metaplasia, squamous metaplasia, and basal cell hyperplasia. Such changes profoundly affect the airway epithelial responses to rhinovirus infection. Previously, we have demonstrated that mucociliary-differentiated cell cultures, established from airway basal cells isolated from COPD patients, show goblet cell and basal cell hyperplasia similar to that observed in patients. These cultures also show a pro-inflammatory phenotype and abnormal innate immune responses to rhinovirus infection. We describe a culturing method that maintains these in vivo features.

Key words Chronic obstructive pulmonary disease, Airway basal cells, Mucociliary differentiation, Innate immunity

1 Introduction

Airway epithelium, a first line of defense, plays a pivotal role in protecting the lungs from environmental insults and orchestrates both innate and adaptive immune responses of the lung to environmental insults. The airway epithelium is pseudostratified and primarily consists of ciliated cells interspersed with goblet cells and Club cells on the luminal side. The basal cells are below the luminal cells and close to the basement membrane. The basal cells are the tissue-specific stem cells and can regenerate fully functional airway epithelium following injury [1]. The airway basal cells can be cultured in vitro at the air/liquid interface to establish mucociliary-differentiated airway epithelium, which closely resembles ciliated cells, goblet cells, club cells, and basal cells [2–5]. These mucociliary-differentiated cultures are extremely useful

Umadevi Sajjan (ed.), *Rhinovirus: Methods and Protocols*, Methods in Molecular Biology, vol. 2903,
https://doi.org/10.1007/978-1-0716-4410-2_9,

models for investigating the innate immune response to infections or other environmental stimuli.

The airway basal cells in patients with chronic lung disease may acquire epigenetic changes due to persistent exposure to the inflammatory milieu, and this can affect their capacity to repair and regenerate airway epithelium. The airway epithelial remodeling, such as goblet cell and squamous metaplasia and basal cell hyperplasia, that is often in patients with chronic obstructive pulmonary disease (COPD), asthma, and cystic fibrosis may reflect impaired epithelial repair by basal cells with acquired epigenetic changes [6–10]. Previously, we have demonstrated that airway basal cells obtained from COPD and cystic fibrosis patients regenerate abnormal airway epithelium with goblet and basal cell hyperplasia when cultured at air/liquid interface [4, 11–13], resembling the features of airway epithelium of patients. COPD cell cultures also express higher levels of pro-inflammatory cytokines than normal cell cultures under basal or unstimulated conditions. COPD cell cultures show exaggerated cytokine and chemokine responses to rhinovirus infection [4, 11, 14]. Maintenance of in vivo features depends on culturing conditions such as passage number of the basal cells, medium used, etc. Here, we describe a modified method of Fulcher et al. [2] to maintain the in vivo features of regenerated airway epithelium from airway basal cells of COPD patients.

2 Materials

1. Tracheobronchial segments from healthy non-smokers can be obtained from lungs rejected for transplantation through non-profit organizations that provide human biomaterial for research (e.g., National Disease Research Interchange www.ndri.com). Tissues from COPD patients can be isolated from explanted lungs or during autopsy through collaboration with surgeons or pathologists. In some cases, it can also be obtained through biobanks that supply fresh tissue specimens. The transport medium used is RPMI medium amended with 100 U/mL of penicillin, 100 μg/mL of streptomycin, and 0.25 μg/mL of amphotericin. The tissues can be stored in the transportation medium for up to 24 h at 4 °C (*see* **Note 1**).
2. Tissue soaking medium: Minimal essential medium (MEM) containing 100 U/mL of penicillin and 100 μg/mL of streptomycin, 0.25 μg/mL of amphotericin +50 μg/mL of gentamycin or tobramycin.
3. Tissue digestion buffer for isolation of airway basal cells contains 1% protease XIV + 0.01% DNase +100 U/mL of penicillin and 100 μg/mL of streptomycin, 0.25 μg/mL of

amphotericin +50 μg/mL of gentamycin or 80 μg/mL of tobramycin in MEM.

4. BronchialLife medium (Lifeline Technologies Cat# LL0023).
5. LHC Basal medium (ThermoFisher Scientific Cat# 12677019).
6. DMEM, high glucose, pyruvate (ThermoFisher Scientific Cat# 11995065).
7. Bovine pituitary extract: Bovine pituitaries (Pel-Freeze Biologicals, Cat# 57133-2). Work in the hood to prepare bovine pituitary extract. We usually prepare extracts from 10 to 15 pituitaries, which will give approximately 50 mL of extract with 13 mg of total protein/mL. Determine the weight of frozen pituitaries. Cut the frozen bovine pituitaries into small pieces. If there are any visible blood clots, remove them with sterile forceps. Suspend pieces of pituitaries in sterile D-PBS without calcium and magnesium two to three times. Finally, suspend the pituitaries at 1 g/1.5 mL of cold D-PBS and grind using a waring blender at 4 °C at high speed for 1 min. Let the homogenate cool for 5–10 min. Repeat the homogenization for another minute. Repeat cooling and homogenization for 1 or more 2 cycles. Centrifuge the homogenate at 4 °C, 2000× *g* for 30 min. Collect the supernatant and subject it to ultracentrifugation at 4 °C, 32,000× *g* for 90 min. Collect the supernatant, and filter through a 0.45 μ filter unit. Using a glass fiber prefilter on top of the filter is recommended to prevent clogging of the membrane. Measure the total protein and store it in the appropriate aliquot sizes at −80 °C. The total protein should be approximately 13 mg/mL.
8. 200× BSA: Tissue culture-grade bovine serum albumin (Millipore Sigma, Cat# A9418). To 10 g of BSA, add 80 mL of PBS, gently rock or leave it at 4 °C overnight. Make up the volume to 100 mL and store in aliquots at −20 °C.
9. 2000× Human Holo Transferrin (Millipore Sigma, Cat# T0665). Dissolve 100 mg of transferrin in 5 ml sterile PBS and store in aliquots at −80 °C.
10. 2000× Insulin from bovine pancreas (Millipore Sigma, Cat# I16634). (10 mg/mL). Dissolve 10 mg of insulin in 200 μL of acetic acid (which will take 5 min at room temperature) and immediately add 4 mL of PBS, store in aliquots at −80 °C.
11. 10,000× Water-soluble hydrocortisone (Millipore Sigma, Cat# H0396). The amount of hydrocortisone in the product varies from batch to batch. Weigh out the product equivalent to 10 mg of hydrocortisone and dissolve in 10 mL of sterile water. Store in aliquots at −80 °C.

12. 2000× All-trans Retinoic acid (Millipore Sigma, Cat# R2625) (RA). Prepare concentrated stock, that is, 1×10^{-3} M RA in 100% ethanol. Dissolve 12 mg of RA in 40 mL of 100% ethanol. Store at −20 °C in 50 mL conical tube wrapped in aluminum foil. To prepare 2000×, dilute the stock 1:100 in ethanol and measure absorbance at 350 nm using a 1 cm light path quartz cuvette against a 100% pure ethanol blank. The diluted stock should have an absorbance ≥0.45. If the absorbance is less than 0.18, discard and prepare fresh. If the OD_{350} is 0.45, then add to 1 mL of 1×10^{-3} M of RA to 1.2 mL of 200× BSA and 7.8 mL of PBS. Keep the RA in aluminum-wrapped tubes all the time. Store these stocks at −80 °C. If the OD_{350} is less or more than 0.45, then adjust the volume of RA accordingly.
13. 10,000× 3,3′,5-Triiodo-L-thyronine sodium salt (T3) (Millipore Sigma, Cat# T6397). Prepare a concentrated stock that is 1 mM T3 by dissolving 6.7 mg in 10 mL of 1 mM NaOH. Dilute 1 mL of 1 mM T3 to 10 mL of 1 mM NaOH and store at −80 °C. Store the concentrated stocks in aliquots at −80 °C.
14. 10,000× Epinephrine (Millipore Sigma, Cat# T4642). Dissolve 44 mg of epinephrine in 10 mL of 0.01 N HCl and store in aliquots at −80 °C.
15. 10,000× O-Phosphorylethanolamine (Millipore Sigma, Cat# P0503). Dissolve 7 mg of O-Phosphorylethanolamine in 10 mL of PBS and store in aliquots at −80 °C.
16. 10,000× Ethanolamine (Millipore Sigma, Cat# E0135, supplied as14.5 M). Dilute 3.4 ul to 10 mL in PBS and store in aliquots at −80 °C.
17. Human Epidermal growth factor, PeproTech (ThermoFisher Scientific, Cat# AF-100-15). Prepare 100 μg/mL in sterile water and store at −80 °C.
18. 1000× Rock Inhibitor Y-27632 Dihydrochloride (Tocris, Cat# 1254). Prepare a concentrated stock of 50 mM Y-27632 in DMSO, dilute to 5 mM in PBS, filter sterilize, and store in aliquots at −20 °C.
19. 1000× calcium chloride: Prepare 0.89 M Calcium chloride in distilled water.
20. 10,000× zinc sulfate (Millipore Sigma Z0251): Prepare 30 mM Zinc sulfate in water.
21. 1000× Stock 4 salt solution: Dissolve 0.42 g of ferrous sulfate (Millipore Sigma, cat# F8048), 122.0 g magnesium chloride hexahydrate (Millipore Sigma, cat# M0250), 16.17 g of calcium chloride dihydrate (Millipore Sigma, cat# C3881), and 5.0 mL of HCl to 800 mL of distilled water. Make up the

volume to 1 L in a volumetric flask and store at room temperature.

22. 1000× trace elements: Prepare the following salt solutions separately. Use a volumetric flask to prepare the salt solutions in distilled water. Fill 500 mL volumetric flask to 100 mL mark, and remove 4 mL of water. Add 0.5 mL of each salt solution and 0.5 mL HCl mix and store at room temperature.

    Trace element stocks.

Salt	Millipore sigma	Molarity	mg/ 100 mL
Sodium selenite	S5261	30.0 mM	518.8
Sodium metasilicate nonahydrate	S5904	500 mM	14,210
Manganese(II) chloride tetrahydrate	M5005	1.0 mM	20
Ammonium molybdate tetrahydrate	M1019	1.0 mM	123.6
Ammonium metavanadate	10,028	5.0 mM	58.5
Nickel(II) sulfate hexahydrate	N4882	1.0 mM	26.3
Tin(II) chloride dihydrate	S9262	500 μM	11.3

23. Growth medium for expanding airway basal cells:
    (a) 500 mL BronchialLife medium + all the additives except for gentamicin and amphotericin.
    (b) EGF 10 μL of 100 μg/mL stock.
    (c) 50 μL of 10,000× all-trans-retinoic acid.
    (d) 50 μL of 5 mM Rock inhibitor Y-27632 (add fresh to the medium on the day of use).
    (e) 100 U/mL of penicillin and 100 μg/mL of streptomycin.
    (f) Additional antibiotics as needed 0.25 μg/mL amphotericin, 50 μg/mL gentamycin or tobramycin, and Nystatin 100 U/mL.

    The medium is stable for up to 3 months. Aliquot the required amount of medium and warm it up to 37 °C just before use. Avoid repeated warming up of the medium to prevent the inactivation of components.

24. Differentiation medium:
    (a) 250 mL of DMEM +250 mL of LHC basal medium
    (b) 5 mL Pen/strep
    (c) 0.5 mL 1000× Trace elements Stock 4 salt solution
    (d) 0.5 mL 1000× Calcium chloride

(e) 2.5 mL 200× Bovine serum albumin
(f) 4 mL BPE (13 mg of total protein/mL)
(g) 0.25 mL 2000× Insulin
(h) 0.25 mL of 2000× Transferrin
(i) 0.25 mL of 2000× Retinoic acid
(j) 20 μL of 100 μg/mL EGF
(k) 50 μL of 10,000× Hydrocortisone
(l) 50 μL of 10,000× Epinephrine
(m) 50 μL of 10,000× O-phosphoryl ethanolamine
(n) 50 μL of 10,000× Ethanolamine
(o) 50 μL of 10,000× Zinc chloride

Filter sterilize using a 0.22 μ filter unit and store at 4 °C. The medium is stable for up to 3 months. Aliquot the required amount of medium and warm it up to 37 °C just before use. Avoid repeated warming up of the medium to prevent the inactivation of components.

25. Declumping reagent: 2 mM EDTA, 0.05 mg/mL DTT, 0.25 mg/mL collagenase, 0.75 mg/mL calcium chloride, 1 mg/mL magnesium chloride, and 10 μg/mL DNase in PBS. Sterile, filter, and store at −20 °C. An alternative to homemade declumping reagent is Accumax from Innovative Cell Technologies (Cat# AM105).
26. Trypsin/EDTA (ThermoFisher Scientific Cat# 25200056). Dilute 20 mL trypsin/EDTA to 50 mL and add 0.5 mL of 500 mM EDTA.
27. Fetal bovine serum.
28. Type I/III collagen: PureCol™ (Advanced Biomatrix).
29. 2× Cell freezing solution: Bronchial epithelial cell growth medium containing 20% FBS and 20% DMSO.
30. Cryovials.
31. Nalgene Cryo Freezing container.
32. Sterile scalpel, scissors, and forceps.
33. 0.4 μ pore size transwells 6.5- or 12-mm wells with PET membrane (Corning Cat# 3470 or 3460) (*see* Fig. 1).
34. 10 and 150 cm cell culture dishes.
35. Rhinovirus.
36. IL-8 and IFN-L1 ELISA kit.
37. AlexaFluor 488-labeled acetylated tubulin antibody.
38. AlexaFluor 594-labeled MUC5B/MUC5AC antibodies.

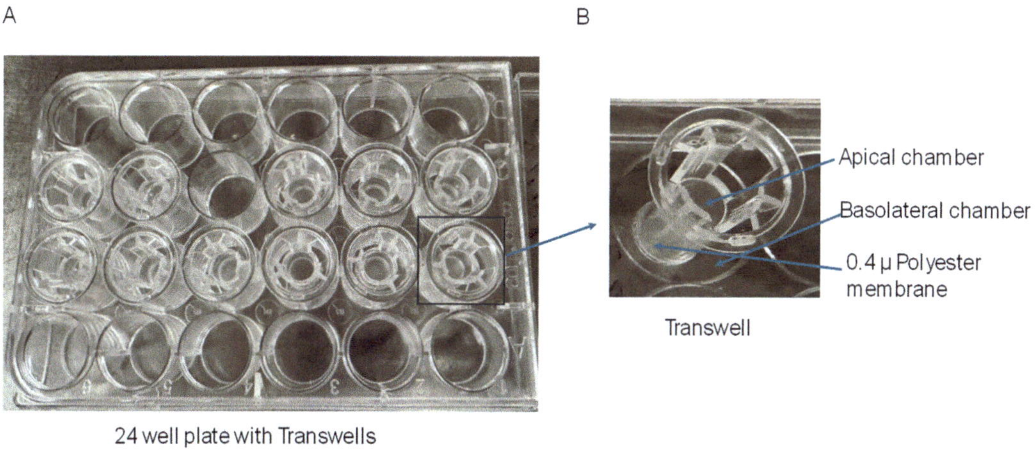

Fig. 1 Transwells purchased from Costar/Corning with polyester membrane. Panel B is the enlarged area marked in Panel A showing transwell

3 Methods

3.1 Isolation of Airway Basal Cells

1. Tissue processing should be performed in the BSL2 biosafety hood: Line the cell culture hood with an absorbent sterile pad. Transfer the tissue to a 150 mm dish. Dissect the airways up to the third branching of the bronchi. Remove connective tissue and lymph nodes. Cut the tissue into 5 × 5 cm pieces and transfer to tissue wash buffer in a sterile conical tube. The ratio of tissue to wash buffer (V/V) should be at least 1:4. Incubate tissue pieces in the wash buffer for 15 min. Transfer the tissue pieces to fresh wash buffer and incubate again for another 15 min.
2. If the tissue has excessive mucus, soak the tissue in soaking buffer for 30 min. Wash the tissue pieces with at least 3 changes of PBS.
3. Transfer tissue pieces to tissue digestion buffer. The ratio of tissue to buffer should be at least 1:3 (V/V).
4. Incubate tissue in digestion buffer for 24 h at 4 °C on a rocker. Add FBS to 10% and mix to neutralize the protease.
5. Transfer the tissue pieces to a 150 mm culture dish containing PBS. Gently scrape the mucosal side of the tissue pieces with the blunt edge of the scalpel to release the epithelial sheets. Collect the scrapings along with the buffer and repeat this scarping process one more time. Combine the scrapings and centrifuge at 4 °C, 1000× g for 10 min.
6. Suspend the cell pellet in the declumping solution and incubate for 15 min to 1 h monitoring the dissociation of clumps (*see* **Note 2**).

7. If using Accumax, mix the cell pellet with Accumax in the ratio of 1:2 and incubate up to 1 h at room temperature. Monitor the cells as in **step 6**.
8. Add FBS to 10% and centrifuge at 500× *g* for 10 min at 4 °C.
9. If using Accumax, dilute the cell/accumax mix by five-fold in PBS with no calcium and magnesium and centrifuge at 500× *g* for 10 min at 4 °C.
10. Suspend the cell pellet in BEGM and count the cells using a hemocytometer. Adjust the density of the cells to at least 2×10^6 cells per mL. Mix 1:1 with cryopreservation medium aliquot 1–1.5 mL into cryovials and transfer cryo freesing container and store and −80 °C for 24 h and then store the cells to liquid phase the nitrogen (*see* **Note 3**).

3.2 Collagen Coating of 10 Cm Dishes and Transwells

1. Add 7 mL of type I/III collagen diluted in water at 5 μg/cm^2 to 10 cm dishes. Incubate overnight at 4 °C. Next day aspirate the remaining solution and dry the plates under UV light in biosafety hood. The plates can be stored at 4 °C for up to 2 months. For storing the plates wrap the plates in saran wrap.
2. Transwells: Dilute PureCol 1:30 with distilled water, add 50 and 100 μL into 6 mm and 12 mm transwell inserts respectively. The transwell inserts should remain in the receiver plates. Incubate overnight at 4 °C. Next day aspirate the remaining solution and dry the transwells under UV light in biosafety hood. The transwells in the receiver plates can be stored at 4 °C for up to 1 month. For storing the plates wrap the plates in saran wrap.

3.3 Culturing the Cells on a 10 Cm Dish

1. Seed freshly isolated P0 or cryopreserved cells on a collagen-coated 10 cm dish. Change the medium every day for the first 3 days (*see* **Note 4**). Then change the medium once in 2 days until the cells become 70–80% confluency (*see* **Note 5**).
2. To detach the cells from the plates, aspirate the medium, rinse twice with PBS, and then add 5 mL diluted cold Trypsin/EDTA. Incubate at 37 °C for 2–3 min. Monitor under the microscope; at this time, the cells should be rounded but not detached.
3. Remove 3 mL of Trypsin/EDTA and continue incubation for an additional 4 min. Never exceed a total of 7 min (*see* **Note 6**).
4. Gently tap the plate against the palm to release the cells from the plate. Add 0.5 mL of FBS to neutralize trypsin and transfer the detached cells to a 50 mL conical tube. Rinse the plate with 10 mL PBS and combine with collected cells.
5. Centrifuge at 500 × g for 5 min at 4 °C, suspend the cells in BEGM, and count the cells. These are P1 cells (*see* **Note 7**).

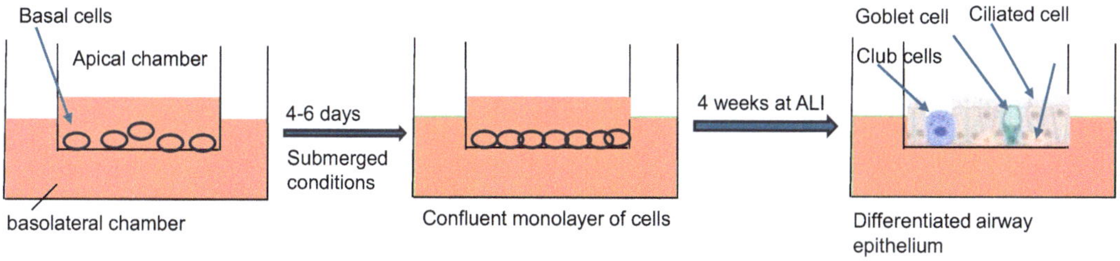

Fig. 2 Steps involved in culturing of airway basal cells. Basal cells at passage 1 are seeded in transwell and grown under submerged conditions using BEGM for 4–6 days or until the cells reach 100% confluence. The cells are then cultured at air/liquid interface in differentiation medium for 4 weeks to promote differentiation into the mucociliary phenotype

3.4 Culturing the Cells in Tanswells to Obtain Mucociliary-Differentiated Airway Epithelium

P1 cells generated from COPD basal cells maintain the acquired epigenetic changes. These epigenetic changes are erased with each passage, and may show similar responses as normal cells. Moreover, normal basal cells at passage 3 and above show more goblet cells than ciliated cells similar to COPD cells. Because of this reason, we use regenerated airway epithelium from P1 cells to determine the differences between COPD and normal cells. The cells cultured on 6.5 mm transwells are better suited for the determination of the morphology of the cultures by histochemistry. The cells cultured on 12 mm transwells can be used for functional studies since there are more cells to get a sufficient amount of total RNA or protein.

1. Seed the P1 cells at a density of 40,000 cells/well for 6.5 mm transwells and 80,000 cells/well for 12 mm transwells (Fig. 2).
2. Add BEGM to both apical and basolateral chambers to culture the cells under submerged conditions until the cells become 100% confluent. It normally takes 4–6 days. Change the medium every 2 days.
3. Remove the medium from the apical chamber to create an air/liquid interface (ALI). For the first 2 days of ALI, feed the cells with BEGM + ALI medium mixed in a 70:30 ratio and the next 2 days with a 50:50 ratio, then for 3 days at a 30: 70 ratio and finally with ALI medium alone.
4. Maintain the cultures in ALI medium for an additional 3 weeks. Change the medium every 2–3 days and remove any medium that is seeped into the apical chamber at the initial stages of ALI culturing.
5. At 3 weeks of culturing at ALI, the cells will start secreting the mucus from the apical surface. The mucus should be removed with a pipette taking care not to injure the epithelial cells. Failure to remove the mucus will lead to dedifferentiation of cultures.

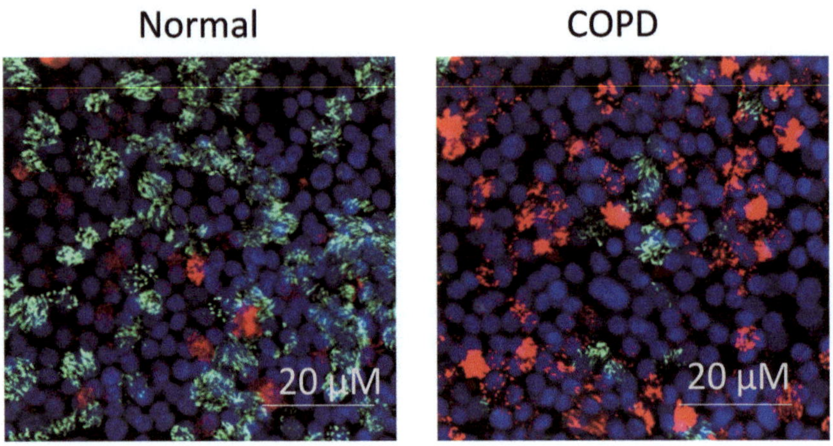

Fig. 3 Normal and COPD basal cells at P1 were cultured at air/liquid interface for 4 weeks. The cells were fixed in cold methanol and immunostained with antibodies to acetylated tubulin (green) to detect cilia and mixture of MUC5B and MUC5AC (red) to detect goblet cells

3.5 Determination of Mucociliary Differentiation of Cultures

1. Wash the cultures from both the apical and basolateral sides with PBS.
2. Add ice-cold methanol to both apical and basolateral chambers and incubate at −20 °C for 5 min.
3. Wash with PBS three times × 5 min.
4. Add PBS containing 1% BSA and incubate for 1 h at room temperature.
5. Incubate with a mixture of acetylated tubulin and MUC5B and/or MUC5AC antibodies for 1 h at room temperature.
6. Wash the cell cultures with PBS three times.
7. Counterstain with DAPI and observe under a fluorescence microscope. The normal cell cultures show an abundant number of ciliated cells with few goblet cells. Whereas COPD cells show fewer ciliated cells and more goblet cells (Fig. 3) (*see* **Note 8**).

3.6 Infection with RV16 and Determination of RV-Stimulated IL-8 and IFN-L1 Responses

1. The steps involved in the infection of airway epithelial cell cultures are outlined in Fig. 4.
2. On the day of infection, rinse the apical surface of the cultures with D-PBS to remove the secreted mucus.
3. Transfer the transwells to a new receiver plate containing fresh ALI medium.
4. Add virus at a multiplicity of infection 1 (3×10^5 virions) in 10 μL to the apical surface (if using 6.5 mm transwells). The control wells should be infected with the same volume of sham [4] (*see* **Note 9**).

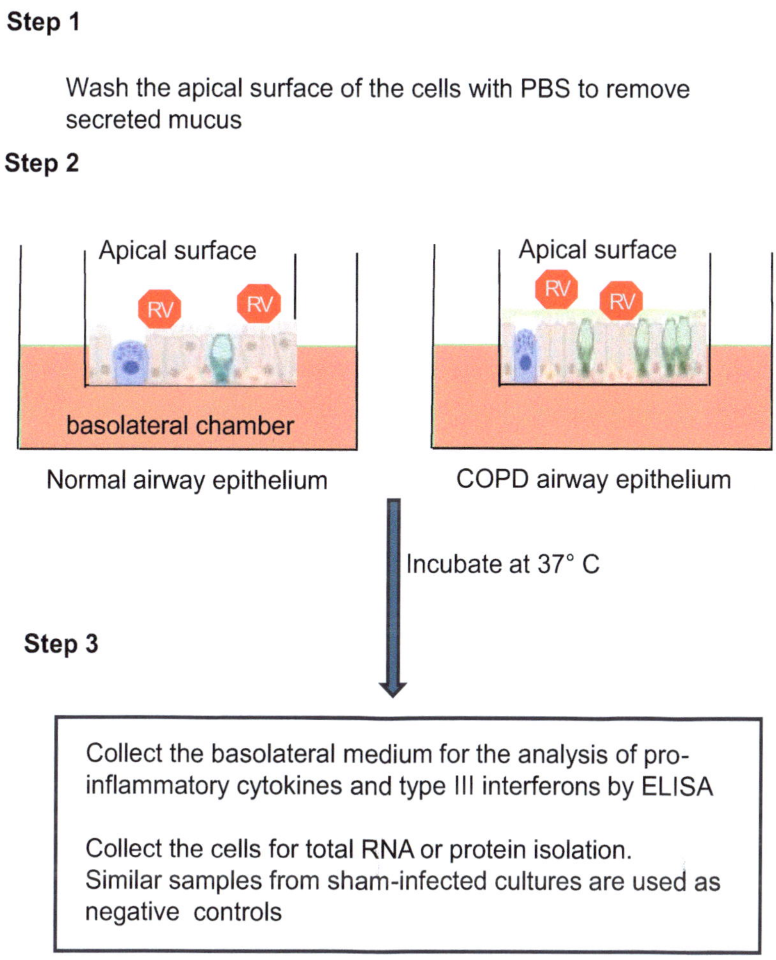

Fig. 4 Infection of airway epithelial cell cultures. Wash the apical surface of the mucociliary-differentiated airway epithelial cell cultures with PBS to remove the secreted mucus. Transfer the transwells to a new receiver plate. Infect the apical surface of the cell cultures with RV or sham (10 uL for 6.5 mm transwells and 30 uL for 12 mm transwells). Incubate for 24 h at 37 °C. Collect the basolateral medium for determination ELISA. Wash the cells with PBS from both the basolateral and apical surfaces of the cell cultures, and add TRIZOL or RIPA buffer directly to the apical surface to collect the lysates for further analysis

5. Incubate for 24 h at 37 °C. Collect the basolateral medium and measure the pro-inflammatory cytokines and type I interferon, IFN-β, and IFN-λ_1.
6. Wash the cells with PBS, lyse cells in TRIZOL, and extract RNA using the Directzol kit and determine the viral RNA by qPCR [16].
7. Results from our study using cells from 8 normal and 8 COPD patients infected with sham or RV are shown in Fig. 5.
8. Compared to normal, COPD cells produce more IL-8 (compared to sham-infected normal and COPD cells), which further increases with RV infection.

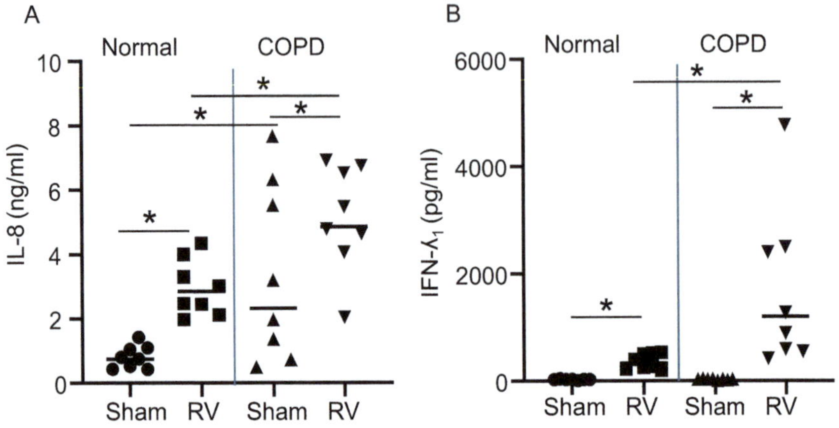

Fig. 5 Levels of IL-8 and IFN-λ_1 in sham and RV-infected normal and COPD cells. Twenty-four hours after the infection, basolateral medium was collected, and the levels of IL-8 and IFN-λ_1 were measured by ELISA ($n = 8$, cells were obtained from 8 normal and 8 COPD patients, $p \leq 0.05$, ANOVA on Ranks)

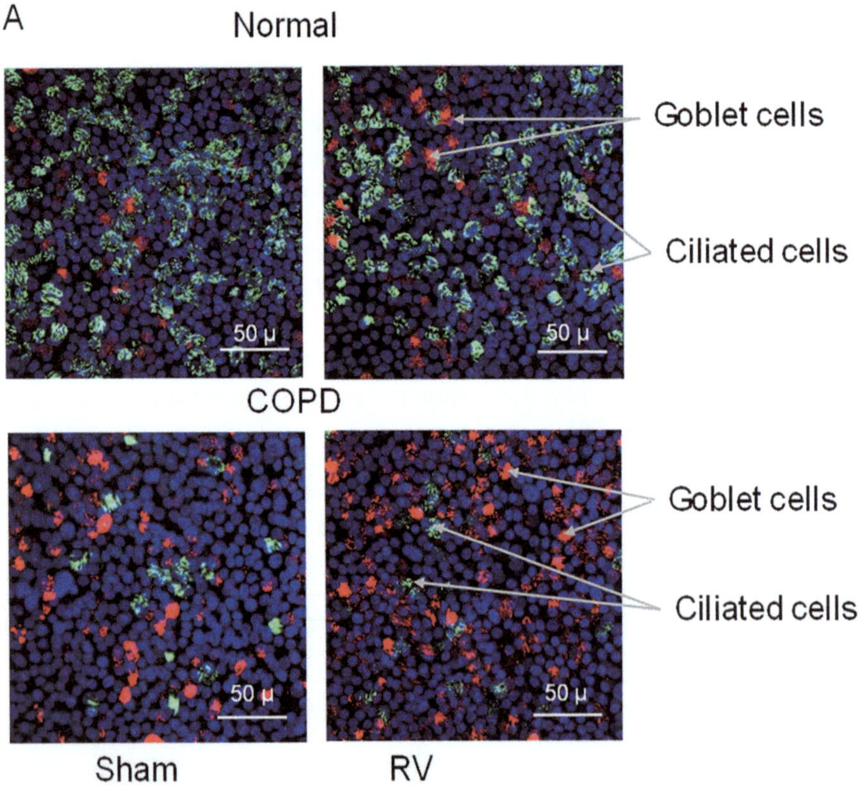

Fig. 6 RV-infected COPD cells show an increase in the number of goblet cells. Normal and COPD cells were infected with sham or RV. The cultures were maintained for 15 days at 37 °C. The cell cultures were fixed and immunostained with antibodies to human tracheobronchial mucins and acetylated tubulin. The bound antibodies were detected by antimouse IgG conjugated with AF 488 (cilia) and antirabbit IgG conjugated with AF 594 (goblet cells). The nuclei were counterstained with DAPI

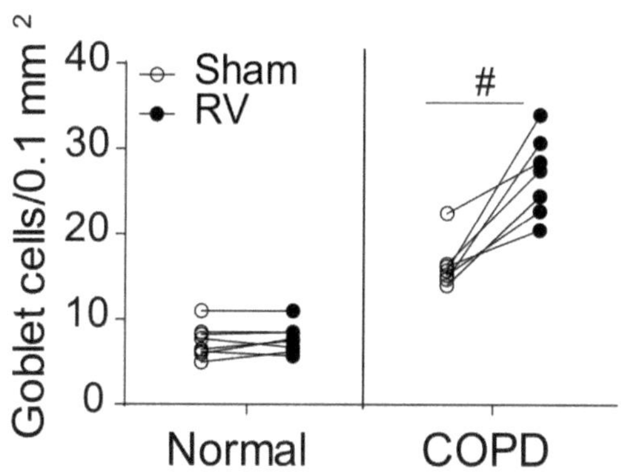

Fig. 7 Quantification of the number of goblet cells in sham- or RV-infected cell cultures. The number of goblet cells was quantified by counting the number of goblet cells per 0.1 mm2 in 5 random fields per image. Data represent intracomparison between sham- and RV-infected 6 7 normal and 7 COPD cell cultures. The paired comparison was conducted by signed rank test (# $p \leq 0.05$)

9. In contrast, there was no difference in the levels of IFN-λ1 in sham-infected cultures between COPD and normal cells. Both normal and COPD cells infected with RV show a significant increase in antiviral IFN response, but it was much higher in COPD than in normal.
10. Since RV does cause minimal cell death, the infected cultures can be maintained for longer periods to examine the long-term effects of RV on the cell cultures.
11. For long-term studies, wash the apical surface of the cell cultures and change the medium in the basolateral chamber every other day.
12. In our studies, we maintained the infected cells for 15 days and examined the cultures for goblet cell metaplasia by staining the cells as described in Subheading 3.5 (Fig. 6a, b).
13. Goblet cells were quantified by counting the cells in 0.1 mm^2 (Fig. 7).
14. Normal cells showed no change in the goblet cell number. In contrast, COPD cells which have goblet cell hyperplasia showed a further increase in goblet cell number, indicating RV increases goblet cells in COPD, but not in normal cultures.

The cells cultured at P1 clearly show a difference between normal and COPD cell cultures in their morphology and responses to rhinovirus infection. COPD cells show goblet cell hyperplasia and produce higher than normal IL-8 under unstimulated conditions, which further increases following RV infection. The COPD cultures infected with RV and maintained for 15 days show a further increase in goblet cells. Similar to our observations in vitro, COPD patients experimentally infected with RV show increased and prolonged pro-inflammatory responses compared to healthy non-smokers [16]. Similarly, we have observed an increase in lung inflammation and goblet cell metaplasia following RV infection in a mouse model of COPD [11, 14, 15]. Based on these observations [11, 14, 15, 16], we recommend the culturing conditions presented in this report will generate the airway epithelium that is structurally similar to in vivo conditions and therefore useful for studying the innate immune responses to viral infection.

4 Notes

1. The donor tissue will have yeast, bacteria, and fungi, and therefore processing the tissue as soon as possible is recommended to prevent overgrowth of these microorganisms and possible carryover to isolated airway basal cells.
2. Accumax can also be used instead of homemade declumping buffer.
3. Storing the cells at less than 1×10^6 cells/mL reduces the viability of cells during storage and thawing.
4. If the cells have contamination, extra antibiotics and antifungal agents can be added to the medium, such as nyostatin (100 U/mL), vancomycin (100 μg/mL), and ceftazidime (100 μg/mL) for the first 3 days. Slowly reduce the antibiotics after 3 days. Primocin (Invivogen), a mixture of antifungal and antibiotics, may also be used instead of single agents separately.
5. Adding Rho kinase inhibitor and SMAD inhibitor promotes the proliferation of airway basal cells, but they also change the epigenetically acquired feature of COPD airway basal cells. Therefore we don't add these inhibitors to the medium.
6. Instead of Trypsin/EDTA accutase, which is gentler and does not neutralize with FBS, it may be used to detach the cells from the plate.
7. If pure airway basal cells are needed, the P1 cells can be selected on NGFR positivity by flow sorting.
8. The COPD basal cells were obtained from patients at end-stage lung disease. The basal cells isolated from mild to moderate COPD patients may show relatively more ciliated cells and fewer goblet cells than the cells from severe COPD patients.
9. It is very important to use very small volumes for infection that is 10 μL for 6.5 mm transwells and 30 μL for 12 mm transwells. Flooding of the surface with higher volume will result in the initiation of dedifferentiation and sloughing of the cells.

References

1. Rock JR, Onaitis MW, Rawlins EL, Lu Y, Clark CP, Xue Y, Randell SH, Hogan BL (2009) Basal cells as stem cells of the mouse trachea and human airway epithelium. Proc Natl Acad Sci USA 106:12771–12775
2. Fulcher ML, Gabriel S, Burns KA, Yankaskas JR, Randell SH (2005) Well-differentiated human airway epithelial cell cultures. Methods Mol Med 107:183–206
3. Sajjan U, Wang Q, Zhao Y, Gruenert DC, Hershenson MB (2008) Rhinovirus disrupts the barrier function of polarized airway epithelial cells. Am J Respir Crit Care Med 178: 1271–1281
4. Schneider D, Ganesan S, Comstock AT, Meldrum CA, Mahidhara R, Goldsmith AM, Curtis JL, Martinez FJ, Hershenson MB, Sajjan U (2010) Increased cytokine response of rhinovirus-infected airway epithelial cells in chronic obstructive pulmonary disease. Am J Respir Crit Care Med 182:332–340
5. Neuberger T, Burton B, Clark H, Van Goor F (2011) Use of primary cultures of human bronchial epithelial cells isolated from cystic fibrosis patients for the pre-clinical testing of CFTR modulators. Methods Mol Biol 741:39–54
6. Rock JR, Randell SH, Hogan BL (2010) Airway basal stem cells: a perspective on their roles in epithelial homeostasis and remodeling. Dis Model Mech 3:545–556
7. Heijink IH, Kuchibhotla VNS, Roffel MP, Maes T, Knight DA, Sayers I, Nawijn MC (2020) Epithelial cell dysfunction, a major driver of asthma development. Allergy 75: 1902–1917
8. Conese M, Di Gioia S (2021) Pathophysiology of lung disease and wound repair in cystic fibrosis. Pathophysiology 28:155–188
9. Crystal RG (2014) Airway basal cells. The "smoking gun" of chronic obstructive pulmonary disease. Am J Respir Crit Care Med 190: 1355–1362
10. Rock JR, Hogan BL (2011) Epithelial progenitor cells in lung development, maintenance, repair, and disease. Annu Rev Cell Dev Biol 27:493–512
11. Jing Y, Gimenes JA, Mishra R, Pham D, Comstock AT, Yu D, Sajjan U (2019) NOTCH3 contributes to rhinovirus-induced goblet cell hyperplasia in COPD airway epithelial cells. Thorax 74:18–32
12. Pineau F, Shumyatsky G, Owuor N, Nalamala N, Kotnala S, Bolla S, Marchetti N, Kelsen S, Criner GJ, Sajjan US (2020) Microarray analysis identifies defects in regenerative and immune response pathways in COPD airway basal cells. ERJ Open Res:6
13. Sajjan U, Keshavjee S, Forstner J (2004) Responses of well-differentiated airway epithelial cell cultures from healthy donors and patients with cystic fibrosis to Burkholderia cenocepacia infection. Infect Immun 72: 4188–4199
14. Ganesan S, Unger BL, Comstock AT, Angel KA, Mancuso P, Martinez FJ, Sajjan US (2013) Aberrantly activated EGFR contributes to enhanced IL-8 expression in COPD airways epithelial cells via regulation of nuclear FoxO3A. Thorax 68:131–141
15. Gimenes, JA, Srivastava V, ReddyVari H, Kotanala S, Mishra R, Farazuddin M, Li W, Sajjan US (2019) Rinovirus induces progression of lung disease in a mouse model of COPD via IL-33/ST2 signaling axis. Clin Sci (Lond) 133:983–996
16. Mallia P, Message SD, Gielen V, Contoli M, Gra K, Kebadze T, Aniscenko J, Laza-Stanca V, Edwards MR, Slater L, Pai A, Stanciu LA, Kon OM, Johnson M, Johnston SL (2011) Experimental rhinovirus infection as a human model of chronic obstructive pulmonary disease exacerbation. Am J Respir Crit Care Med 183:734–742

Chapter 10

Investigation of Differentiated Nasal Epithelial Responses to Infection with Clinical Isolates of *Rhinovirus* A and C

Rebecca L. Watkinson, Yury A. Bochkov, James E. Gern, Thomas Iosifidis, Kevin Looi, Ingrid A. Laing, and Anthony Kicic

Abstract

The nasal epithelium is the primary point of contact for inhaled respiratory viruses such as rhinovirus, respiratory syncytial virus, influenza, and coronavirus, among others. In order to establish infection, these viruses must engage their respective receptors located on host epithelial cells and begin replication. However, the nasal epithelium is also a pivotal orchestrator of both structural and innate immune defenses against these pathogens and thus mounts a broad antiviral response to halt the progression of the infection into the lower airways. Of note, the most common virus found in the airways of children presenting to the hospital emergency department with acute wheezing and asthma is *rhinovirus C* (RV-C), followed by *rhinovirus A* (RV-A). Here, we illustrate infection of a preclinical differentiated nasal epithelial model with clinical isolates of RV-A and -C, in conjunction with several methods utilized for characterization of epithelial responses post-infection in vitro.

Key words Nasal epithelium, Rhinovirus, Viral infection, Asthma, Epithelial barrier, Receptors, Cytokines, Confocal microscopy, Pediatrics, Wheeze

1 Introduction

The epithelial cells that line the nasal passages and airways are the first point of contact for many inhaled pathogens. Interactions between respiratory pathogens such as *rhinovirus* (RV), respiratory syncytial virus (RSV), influenza, and coronavirus, and the nasal epithelium are multifaceted. In order to achieve active infection and replicate, these viruses must attach to their respective receptors expressed on the surface of epithelial cells [1–4]. However, the nasal epithelium is not only a conduit of the viral replication cycle but also orchestrates both structural and innate immune defenses and is thus pivotal in maintaining airway homeostasis [5–9]. This is particularly important as the capacity for antiviral defenses in the nasal epithelium may halt the progression of infection into the

Umadevi Sajjan (ed.), *Rhinovirus: Methods and Protocols*, Methods in Molecular Biology, vol. 2903,
https://doi.org/10.1007/978-1-0716-4410-2_10,

lower airways that could result in heightened immune responses [10].

Viral infections commonly lead to acute wheezing in children, which is associated with the development of asthma [11–13]. The most common respiratory virus found in children presenting to the emergency department with acute wheeze and asthma is RV, particularly species C, followed by species A [14–16]. In the community, RV is referred to as one of the viruses that cause the common cold, and it is currently unknown as to why it is associated with acute wheeze and asthma pathology in susceptible children. It is postulated that the prevalence of RV-induced wheeze in the emergency department may be in part due to underlying epithelial vulnerabilities in the airways of children susceptible to recurrent exacerbations and asthma development, highlighting the need for preclinical infection studies [5, 9, 17, 18]. Previously, RV-C15 infection of differentiated healthy adult bronchial epithelial cells was found to elicit epithelial barrier disruption and the release of cytokines, including interleukin (IL) 6, IL8 (CXCL8), RANTES (CCL5), and IP10 (CXCL10) [19], suggesting that these epithelial responses should be investigated in the context of RV infection in pediatric acute wheeze and asthma. In addition, dysregulation has already been elucidated in epithelial responses to infection with RV (RV-A1B) in the bronchial epithelial cells from children with stable asthma compared to children without asthma, such as dissociation and reduction in expression of adherence junctional complex genes and proteins, higher levels of pro-inflammatory and antiviral-specific cytokines IL6, IL8, RANTES, and IP10, lower interferon-beta release, potentiated aberrant cellular repair processes, and less epithelial apoptosis [20–23]. However, potential underlying vulnerabilities and aberrant responses to RV infection in the epithelium of children with acute wheeze and asthma have not yet been investigated, particularly with clinical isolates of RV-A and C found in children. This is because there are limited pediatric-derived nasal epithelial cell models of RV infection, particularly in regard to acutely wheezing children due to the nature of their illness and the need for infection with clinical isolates of RV to better understand the antiviral responses in health and disease.

Here, we describe several methodologies which can be utilized to investigate epithelial responses to clinical isolates of RV-A and C in a differentiated epithelial model derived from a pediatric cohort.

2 Materials

1. *70% (v/v) Ethanol (EtOH)*: Prepare by adding 15 mL absolute EtOH (molecular grade, Sigma-Aldrich, St. Louis, MO, USA) to 35 mL ddH_2O and store at room temperature.

2. *Sterile Phosphate Buffered Saline (PBS)*: Prepare by dissolving 1× PBS tablet (Thermo Fisher Scientific, Waltham, MA, USA) in 500 mL ddH_2O, followed by autoclaving and storing at room temperature.
3. *Non-sterile Phosphate Buffered Saline (PBS)*: Prepare a 10× PBS stock solution by dissolving 80.0 g NaCl, 2.0 g KCl, 14.4 g NaH_2PO_4, and 2.4 g KH_2PO_4 in 1 L of ddH_2O. Adjust pH to 7.4 using a pH meter and calibration solutions prior to storing at room temperature. Dilute to 1× PBS in ddH_2O before use.
4. *HEPES (4-(2-hydroxyethyl)-1-piperazineethanesulphonic acid)—Buffered Hank's Balanced Salt Solution (H-HBSS)*: Prepare by dissolving 8.0 g NaCl, 0.4 g KCl, 0.14 g $CaCl_2$, 0.1 g $MgSO_4.7H_2O$, 0.1 g $MgCl_2.6H_2O$, 0.06 g $Na_2HPO_4.2H_2O$, 0.06 g KH_2PO_4, 1.0 g D-Glucose, 0.35 g $NaHCO_3$, and 5.96 g HEPES (Sigma-Aldrich, St. Louis, MO, USA) in 1 L of ddH_2O. Adjust the pH to 7.4 using a pH meter and calibration solutions. Filter-sterilize and store at 4 °C.
5. *Interleukin (IL) 6 and IL8 Coating Buffer*: Prepare by dissolving 1.59 g Na_2CO_3 and 2.93 g $NaHCO_3$ in 1 L ddH_2O. Adjust the pH to 9.6 with a pH meter and calibration solutions prior to storing at −20 °C.
6. *IL6 Blocking Buffer*: Prepare by dissolving 6.05 g Tris (MW 121.1), 9.0 g Na_2CO_3, and 0.25 g NaN_3 in 800 mL ddH_2O. Add 3.5 mL of 33% HCl and adjust the pH to 7.4 using a pH meter and calibration solutions. Add 5 g of Bovine Serum Albumin (BSA, Sigma-Aldrich, St. Louis, MO, USA) and make sure it has fully dissolved before increasing the final volume to 1 L with ddH_2O. Store at −20 °C.
7. *IL6 TRF Wash Buffer*: Prepare a 10× stock by dissolving 60.5 g Tris (MW 121.1), 90 g NaCl, and 2.5 g NaN_3 in 800 mL ddH_2O. Add 30 mL of 33% HCl and adjust the pH to 7.8 using a pH meter and calibration solutions prior to increasing the final volume to 1 L with ddH_2O. Store at room temperature and dilute the Wash Buffer to a 1× solution in ddH2O and add Tween-20 (Sigma-Aldrich, St. Louis, MO, USA) to a final concentration of 0.05% (v/v) prior to use.
8. *IL8 Wash Buffer*: Add Tween-20 to non-sterile 1× PBS at a final concentration of 0.05% (v/v). Store between 2 °C and 8 °C and use within 3 days.
9. *IL8 Assay Diluent*: Add Fetal Calf Serum (FCS) to non-sterile 1× PBS at a final concentration of 10% (v/v). The pH should be 7.0. Store between 2 °C and 8 °C and use within 7 days.
10. *RANTES (CCL5) and IP10 (CXCL10) ELISA Reagent Diluent*: Add BSA (Sigma-Aldrich, St. Louis, MO, USA) to non-sterile 1× PBS at a final concentration of 1% (w/v). The

pH should be between 7.2 and 7.4. Store between 2 °C and 8 °C and use within 7 days.

11. *RANTES (CCL5) and IP10 (CXCL10) ELISA Wash Buffer*: Prepare by adding Tween-20 (Sigma-Aldrich, St. Louis, MO, USA) to non-sterile 1× PBS at a final concentration of 0.05% (v/v). The pH should be 7.2–7.4. Store at 2–8 °C and use within 3 days.
12. *Tris Buffered Saline (TBS)*: Prepare a 10× stock by dissolving 80 g NaCl, 2 g KCl, and 30 g Trizma Base (Sigma-Aldrich, St. Louis, MO, USA) in 1 L of ddH_2O. Adjust pH to 7.4 using a pH meter and calibration solutions prior to storing at room temperature. Dilute to 1× TBS with ddH_2O prior to use.
13. *Saponin (0.1% w/v)*: Prepare by dissolving saponin (Sigma-Aldrich/Merck, St. Louis, MO, USA) in 1× TBS to a final concentration of 0.1% (w/v). Store at 4 °C until use.
14. *Immunofluorescence (IF) Blocking Buffer*: Add Normal Goat Serum (GIBCO, Waltham, MA, USA) at a final concentration of 10% (v/v), FCS (Life Technologies, Carlsbad, CA, USA) to a final concentration of 10% (v/v), and BSA (Sigma-Aldrich/Merck, St. Louis, MO, USA) to a final concentration of 1% (w/v) in 1× TBS. Store at 2–8 °C.
15. *Triton-×-100 Solution (10% v/v)*: Add 10 mL of Triton-×-100 (Sigma-Aldrich, St. Louis, MO, USA) stock solution to 90 mL of non-sterile 1× PBS and store at room temperature.
16. *Triton-×-100 Permeabilization and Blocking Solution*: Prepare by adding Normal Goat Serum (GIBCO, Waltham, MA, USA) at a final concentration of 10% (v/v) FCS (Life Technologies, Carlsbad, CA, USA) to a final concentration of 10% (v/v) BSA (Sigma-Aldrich/Merck, St. Louis, MO, USA) to a final concentration of 1% (w/v) and Triton-×-100 solution to a final concentration of 1% (v/v) in 1× TBS. Store at 2–8 °C.

3 Methods

3.1 Determination of Viral Titers

Preface: Additional protocols and steps not described in this chapter were carried out to propagate clinical isolates of RV (RV-A16 and RV-C15 that were cloned from the nasopharyngeal aspirate of infected children).

3.1.1 RNA Extraction as Per the PureLink RNA Mini Kit

1. Collect a 10 μL aliquot of purified RV-A16 or RV-C15 progeny virions and add it to 350 μL of RLT lysis buffer (PureLink, Ambion, Life Technologies, Waltham, MA, USA) containing 1% (v/v) β-mercaptoethanol (Qiagen, Hilden, Germany) for capsid and protein lysis.

2. Add an equivalent amount of 70% (v/v) ethanol and pipette repeatedly to mix and disperse any visible precipitate.
3. Transfer the mixture to a spin cartridge (PureLink Life Technologies, Waltham, MA, USA) and centrifuge at 12,000 g for 15 s at room temperature before discarding the flow through.
4. Add 700 μL of Wash Buffer I (PureLink, Ambion, Life Technologies, Waltham, MA, USA) to the spin cartridge and centrifuge at 12,000 g for 15 s at room temperature before discarding flow through.
5. Optional on-column DNase I (PureLink, Ambion, Life Technologies, Waltham, MA, USA) treatment to remove residual DNA is carried out by adding 80 μL of the following mixture to the spin cartridge followed by a 15-min incubation at room temperature.

   DNase Treatment per Column

   - 10× DNase I Reaction Buffer (8 μL)
   - Resuspended 3 U/μL DNase (10 μL).
   - RNase-Free H_2O (62 μL).
6. Add 700 μL of Wash Buffer I (PureLink, Ambion, Life Technologies, Waltham, MA, USA) to the spin cartridge and centrifuge at 12,000 g for 15 s at room temperature before discarding flow through and transferring the column into a new collection tube.
7. Add 500 μL of Wash Buffer II (PureLink, Ambion, Life Technologies, Waltham, MA, USA) to the spin cartridge and centrifuge at 12,000 g for 15 s at room temperature before discarding flow through. Repeat this twice.
8. Dry the spin cartridge membrane by centrifuging at 12,000 g for 2 min at room temperature before transferring it into a recovery tube (PureLink, Ambion, Life Technologies, Waltham, MA, USA).
9. To recover the purified viral RNA, add 30 μL of RNase-free H_2O (Thermo Fisher Scientific, Waltham, MA, USA) to the spin cartridge and incubate for 1 min at room temperature prior to centrifuging at 12,000 g for 2 min at room temperature to elute the RNA.
10. Viral RNA should be stored at −80 °C for future use.

3.1.2 Reverse Transcription of RV-A16 and RV-C15

1. Prepare a reaction mixture containing the following reagents (Thermo Fisher Scientific, Waltham, MA, USA):

   Reaction Volume: 10 μL per virus

   - $MgCl_2$: 2.2 μL.
   - dNTPs: 2 μL,

Table 1
Forward and reverse primer sequences for rhinovirus stock determination by PCR

Primer [Stock]	Sequence	[Final]
RV1A16 Forward[a] [10 μM]	5′- CCTCCGGCCCCTGAAT—3′	0.3 μM/reaction
R848 Reverse[a] [10 μM]	5′- AAACACGGACACCCAAAGTAGT—3′	0.3 μM/reaction

[a]Universal RV Primers (anneal to conserved regions in the 5′UTR of RV, thus are able to amplify all three species, A, B, and C: amplicon size 117 base pairs, Integrated DNA Technologies, Coralville, IA, USA)

- 10× Reverse Transcription Buffer: 1 μL
- R848 Primer (refer to Table 1 for sequence).

  (Integrated DNA Technologies, Coralville, IA, USA): 20 μM, 0.5 μL
- RNase Inhibitor: 0.2 μL.
- MultiScribe Reverse Transcriptase: 0.25 μL.

2. Add 3.85 μL of purified RV-A16 or RV-C15 to the reaction mixture, flicking to mix, followed by centrifugation to collect at the bottom of the tube.
3. Incubate the viral RNA and reaction mixture according to the following parameters prior to diluting the cDNA 1:5 with RNase-free H_2O (Thermo Fisher Scientific, Waltham, MA, USA) and storing at −20 °C until use.

   BioRad ThermoCycler (BioRad, Hercules, CA, USA) parameters for cDNA generation:
   - 30 min at 48 °C
   - 5 min at 95 °C
   - Infinite hold at 4 °C.

3.1.3 Quantitative PCR

1. Prepare a mastermix containing the following reagents:

   Reaction Volume: 10 μL per well required
   - 2× SYBR Green PCR Mix (Thermo Fisher Scientific, Waltham, MA, USA): 5 μL
   - RNase-free H_2O (Thermo Fisher Scientific, Waltham, MA, USA): 2.4 μL
   - Universal RV Primers (refer to Table 1 for forward and reverse sequences).
2. Pipette 8 μL of mastermix into each well required of a 96-well qPCR plate (#HSP9601, BioRad, Hercules, CA, USA).
3. Add 2 μL RNase-free H_2O (Thermo Fisher Scientific, Waltham, MA, USA) into designated wells in duplicate as a non-template control (NTC).

4. To achieve a calculated viral titer for the stock virus, a standard curve generated from ten-fold serially diluted RV cDNA with a known infectious titer (PFU, PFU/mL, RNA copies, copies/mL) is required. Add 2 μL of each dilution in duplicate to designated wells on the qPCR plate as viral titer standards. Alternatively, standards can be generated from full-length in vitro transcribed RV-C15, for which 0.1 μg RNA is approximately equal to 2.62×10^{10} copies of virus.
5. Add 2 μL of the unknown RV-A16 or RV-C15 cDNA in duplicate to designated wells on the qPCR plate. It is optional to include serial dilutions to account for titers that may be higher than the most concentrated standard.
6. Utilizing a CFX96 Touch Real-Time qPCR Detection System (BioRad, Hercules, CA, USA), cycle using the following parameters and capture melt-curve data:
   - 2 min at 50 °C
   - 10 min at 95 °C
   - 15 s at 95 °C (40 cycles)
   - 1 min at 60 °C
7. Check melt-curve analysis to confirm a single peak in the same range as the standards (approximate melt temperature 81 °C). Note: At high cycle thresholds a broad-based melt curve may appear which indicates non-specific amplification rather than low level detection of the virus.
8. Utilizing averaged Ct values, use the linear equation $y = mx + c$ generated with the RV standards to determine Viral Titre $_{\text{Unknown}}$ through the following calculations:
   - $\text{Log[Viral Titre]}_{\text{Unknown}} = (\text{Unknown Titre Ct} - c)/m.$
   - $\text{Viral Titre}_{\text{Unknown}} = 10^{(\text{Log[Viral Titre]Unknown})}.$

3.2 Viral Infection

1. Prepare a viral inoculum by diluting RV-A16 or RV-C15 stock in growth media with 0.01% (w/v) Bovine Serum Albumin (BSA, Sigma-Aldrich, St. Louis, MO, USA) to the desired working concentration [24, 25].
2. Prepare ultraviolet-inactivated viral inoculum by exposing an aliquot of stock virus to UV light for 20 min prior to diluting as per step 1 (shorter exposures to UV light are preferred depending on the intensity of the light source, as long exposures to intense UV light may result in evaporation, protein fragmentation, or RNA nicking). This is utilized to confirm that epithelial responses to RV-A16 or RV-C15 are attributed to active viral infection.
3. Remove the growth media from the basolateral compartment of the differentiated nasal epithelial cell culture and wash the

apical surface three times with sterile 1× PBS to remove excess mucus.

4. Pipette 100 μL of viral inoculum onto the apical surface of the differentiated cell culture and rock plates gently on a shaker for 15 min at room temperature [24, 25].
5. Transfer the plates into a non-shaking incubator with an atmosphere consisting of 95% air and 5% CO_2 at 37 °C for 4 h [24, 25].
6. Aspirate the viral inoculum and wash the apical surface of the differentiated cell culture with sterile 1× PBS to remove excess viral inoculum. The inoculum can also be collected for viral attachment studies by quantifying remaining free virions [24, 25].
7. Restore growth media to the basolateral compartment of the cell culture and incubate further until sample collection at the designated timepoint.

3.3 Viral Load (See *Fig. 1a*)

To detect viral infection and quantify the viral load, the amount of viral RNA is measured by RT-qPCR [26].

3.3.1 RNA Extraction as Per the PureLink RNA Mini Kit

1. Submerge the differentiated nasal epithelial cell culture still attached to the insert membrane into 350 μL of RLT lysis buffer (PureLink, Ambion, Life Technologies, Waltham, MA, USA) containing 1% (v/v) β-mercaptoethanol (Qiagen, Hilden, Germany) to achieve full cell lysis.
2. Add an equivalent amount of 70% (v/v) ethanol and pipette repeatedly to mix and disperse any visible precipitate.
3. Transfer the mixture to a spin cartridge (PureLink Life Technologies, Waltham, MA, USA) and centrifuge at 12,000 *g* for 15 s at room temperature before discarding flow through.
4. Add 700 μL of Wash Buffer I (PureLink, Ambion, Life Technologies, Waltham, MA, USA) to the spin cartridge and centrifuge at 12,000 *g* for 15 s at room temperature before discarding flow through.
5. Optional on-column DNase I (Invitrogen, Thermo Fisher Scientific, Waltham, MA, USA) treatment to remove residual DNA is carried out by adding 80 μL of the following mixture to the spin cartridge followed by a 15-min incubation at room temperature.

   DNase Treatment per Column

   - 10× DNase I Reaction Buffer (8 μL)
   - Resuspended 3 U/μL DNase (10 μL).
   - RNase-Free H_2O (62 μL).

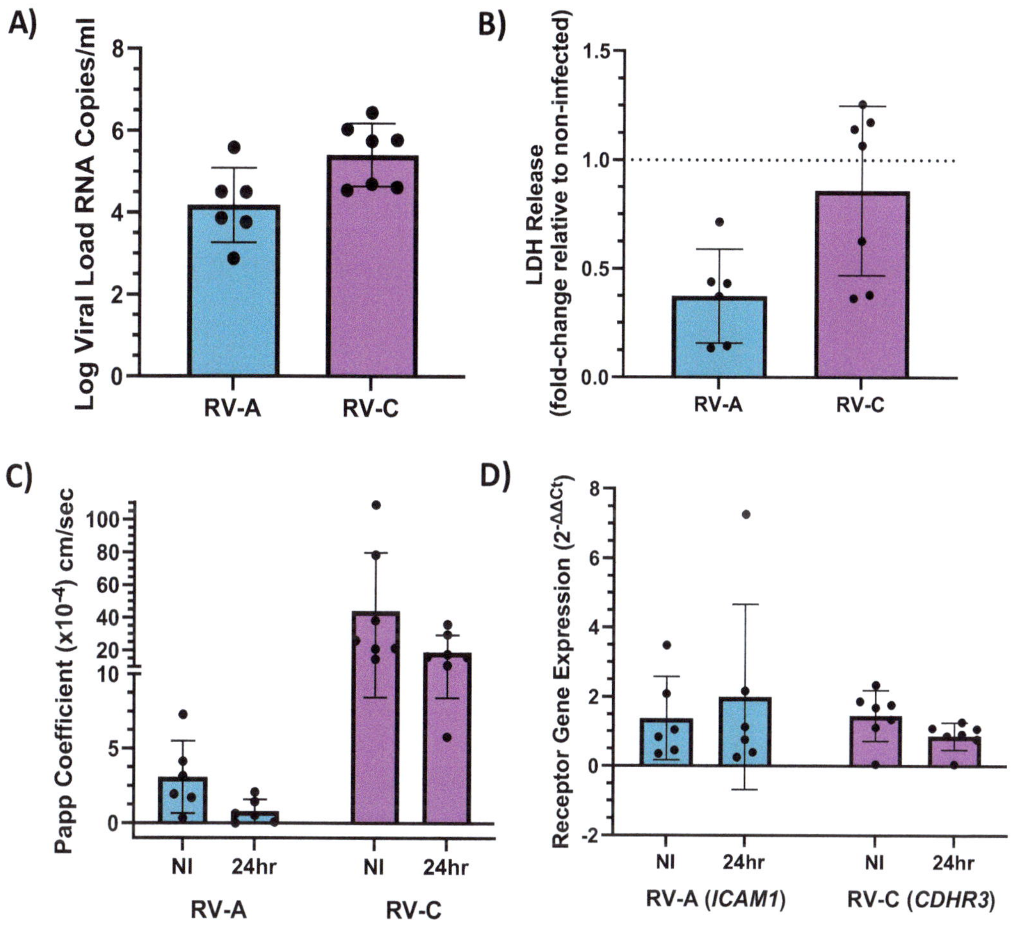

Fig. 1 (**a**) Log viral load at 24 h post-infection with RV-A16 or RV-C15; (**b**) Release of LDH relative to non-infected controls at 24 h post-infection with RV-A16 or RV-C15; (**c**) Epithelial permeability of non-infected NEC cultures (NI) and at 24 h post-infection with RV-A16 or RV-C15; (**d**) Receptor gene expression in non-infected NEC cultures and at 24 h post-infection with RV-A16 (receptor *ICAM1*) or RV-C15 (receptor *CDHR3*). Data points are representative of the assay

6. Add 700 μL of Wash Buffer I (PureLink, Ambion, Life Technologies, Waltham, MA, USA) to the spin cartridge and centrifuge at 12,000 *g* for 15 s at room temperature before discarding flow through and transferring the column into a new collection tube.
7. Add 500 μL of Wash Buffer II (PureLink, Ambion, Life Technologies, Waltham, MA, USA) to the spin cartridge, and centrifuge at 12,000 *g* for 15 s at room temperature before discarding flow through. Repeat this twice.
8. Dry the spin cartridge membrane by centrifuging at 12,000 *g* for 2 min at room temperature before transferring it into a

recovery tube (PureLink, Ambion, Life Technologies, Waltham, MA, USA).

9. To recover the purified epithelial RNA, add 30 μL of RNase-free H_2O (Thermo Fisher Scientific, Waltham, MA, USA): to the spin cartridge and incubate for 1 min at room temperature prior to centrifuging at 12,000 *g* for 2 min at room temperature to elute the RNA.
10. Epithelial RNA should be stored at −80 °C for future use.

3.3.2 Reverse Transcription of Epithelial Culture RNA

1. Prepare a reaction mixture containing the following reagents (Thermo Fisher Scientific, Waltham, MA, USA):
   Reaction Volume: 20 μL per sample
   - $MgCl_2$: [final] 5.5 mM.
   - dNTPs: [final] 0.5 mM per dNTP,
   - 10× Reverse Transcription Buffer:
   - Random Hexamers: [final] 2.5 μM.
   - RNase Inhibitor: (8 U).
   - MultiScribe Reverse Transcriptase (25 U).
2. Add the required volume of 200 ng of purified epithelial RNA to the reaction mixture, flicking to mix, followed by centrifugation to collect at the bottom of the tube.
3. Add the required volume of RNase-free H_2O (Thermo Fisher Scientific, Waltham, MA, USA) to the mixture to bring the volume up to 20 μL.
4. Incubate the epithelial RNA and reaction mixture according to the following parameters prior to diluting the cDNA 1:5 with RNase-free H_2O (Thermo Fisher Scientific, Waltham, MA, USA): and storing at −20 °C until use.
   BioRad ThermoCycler (BioRad, Hercules, CA, USA) parameters for cDNA generation:
   - 10 min at 25 °C
   - 30 min at 48 °C
   - 5 min at 95 °C
   - Infinite hold at 4 °C.

3.3.3 Quantitative PCR: Absolute Quantitation of Viral Load

1. See Subheading 3.1.1. *Quantitative PCR.*

3.4 Cell Death (See Fig. 1b)

To quantify the effect of viral infection on cell viability, the amount of LDH released is measured using the CytoTox96® Non-Radioactive Cytotoxicity Assay (Promega, Madison, WI, USA) [19, 22, 27].

1. Collect supernatant from the basolateral compartment and washes from the apical surface of the differentiated nasal epithelial culture at the experimental designated timepoints and store at −80 until use.
2. Thaw samples and add 25 μL of each to duplicate wells in a 96-well plate (NUNC, Thermo Fisher Scientific, Waltham, MA, USA).
3. Use unused growth media in which the cells were cultured as a blank correction for this assay.
4. Add an equivalent volume of CytoTox96 reagent to each well.
5. Incubate the plate for 30 min at room temperature away from light.
6. Add an equivalent amount of Stop Solution to halt the reaction.
7. Read absorbance on a plate reader at an absorbance of 490 nm.
8. Infected samples can be compared to control samples using fold change increase in LDH, or a positive control of 100% cell lysis can be used to calculate percentage plasma membrane lysis.

3.5 Trans-Epithelial Permeability Assay (See Fig. 1e)

To quantify the effects of viral infection on epithelial barrier, the trans-epithelial permeability assay is used [20, 28].

1. At the designated timepoint post infection, collect the growth media from the basolateral compartment of the differentiated nasal epithelial culture. Washes of the apical surface can be carried out and collected prior to this assay to remove excess mucus and for baseline assessments.
2. To the basolateral compartment of the differentiated epithelial culture, add 1 mL of 1× HEPES-Buffered Hanks Balanced Salt Solution (H-HBSS).
3. Add 200 μL of 4 kDa FITC-Dextran (2 mg/mL w/v in 1× H-HBSS) to the apical surface of the epithelial culture.
4. Collect 50% of the FITC-Dextran from the apical surface and replace. The collected FITC-Dextran will provide an apical timepoint zero for analysis.
5. Collect 50% of the H-HBSS from the basolateral compartment and replace. The collected H-HBSS will provide a blank or basolateral timepoint zero for analysis.
6. Place cultures on an orbital shaker moving at 300 rpm at 37 °C in an atmosphere of 95% air and 5% CO_2.
7. At timepoint 30 min, and then hourly between and inclusive of 1–6 h, collect 50% of the H-HBSS from the basolateral

compartment of the epithelial culture and replace with fresh H-HBSS.

8. Post-assay, aliquot 50 μL of each collected sample into a 96-well plate (Black/Clear Bottom Plates, TC Surface, Thermo Fisher Scientific, Waltham, MA, USA, are preferred to reduce fluorescence bleed-through).
9. Read plates containing the samples on a Plate Reader with an excitation wavelength of 492 nm and an emission of 520 nm.
10. Apparent epithelial paracellular permeability (units P_{app} cm/s) was calculated according to the following equation and parameters [20, 28]:

$$P_{app} = (dQ/dt) \times (1/AC_0)$$

dQ/dt = steady state flux,

A = culture insert surface area.

C_0 = initial concentration.

3.6 Expression of Gene Targets: Viral Receptors (See Fig. 1d)

Here, we describe methods for viral receptor gene expression relative to Peptidylprolyl Isomerase A / Cyclophilin A (PPIA), which has been highlighted as a preferred housekeeping gene for epithelial cells across different cohorts [29].

3.6.1 RNA Extraction

1. See Subheading 3.3. *RNA Extraction as per the PureLink RNA Mini Kit.*

3.6.2 Reverse Transcription PCR

1. See Subheading 3.3. *Reverse Transcription of Epithelial Culture RNA.*

3.6.3 Quantitative PCR: Relative Expression of Gene Targets

1. Prepare a mastermix containing the following reagents:
   Reaction Volume: 10 μL per well required
   - 2× SYBR Green PCR Mix (Thermo Fisher Scientific, Waltham, MA, USA): 5 μL
   - Nuclease-free H_2O (Thermo Fisher Scientific, Waltham, MA, USA): 2.4 μL
   - Forward and Reverse Primers specific to gene target (refer to Table 2 for forward and reverse primers Integrated DNA Technologies, Coralville, IA, USA):
2. Pipette 8 μL of mastermix into each well required of a 96-well qPCR plate (#HSP9601, BioRad, Hercules, CA, USA).
3. Add 2 μL RNase-free H_2O (Thermo Fisher Scientific, Waltham, MA, USA) into designated wells in duplicate as a non-template control (NTC).

Table 2
Forward and reverse primer sequences for relative viral receptor gene expression by PCR

Primer [Stock]	Sequence	[Final]
ICAM1 forward [10 μM]	5′—TATGGCAACGACTCCTTCT—3′	0.3 μM/reaction
ICAM1 reverse [10 μM]	5′—CATTCAGCGTCACCTTGG—3′	0.3 μM/reaction
CDHR3 forward [10 μM]	5′—TGTGAAGGATGAGGTTGGTG—3′	0.3 μM/reaction
CDHR3 reverse [10 μM]	5′—TCCAGGGTTTGCTCTTTCTAC—3′	0.3 μM/reaction
PPIA forward [10 μM]	5′—TGAGCACTGGAGAGAAAGGA—3′	0.3 μM/reaction
PPIA reverse [10 μM]	5′—CCATTATGGCGTGTAAAGTCA—3′	0.3 μM/reaction

4. To test the efficiency of the primers, a standard curve should be generated using five-fold serially diluted standards from samples containing high levels of the target gene. Add 2 μL of each dilution in duplicate to designated wells on the qPCR plate.
5. Add 2 μL of each epithelial culture sample cDNA in duplicate to designated wells on the qPCR plate.
6. Duplicate all wells containing target gene mastermix side by side with separate wells containing PPIA mastermix on the same 96-well qPCR plate (NTC, standards, samples).
7. Utilizing a CFX96 Touch Real-Time qPCR Detection System (BioRad, Hercules, CA, USA), cycle using the following parameters and capturing melt-curve data:
   - 2 min at 50 °C
   - 10 min at 95 °C
   - 15 s at 95 °C (40 cycles)
   - 1 min at 60 °C
8. Check melt-curve analysis to confirm a single peak and no dimerization of primers.
9. Calculate relative gene expression using the delta-delta Ct qPCR method to normalize to the housekeeping gene and endogenous control.

3.7 Cytokine Release

Here, we describe methods to investigate cytokines IL6, IL8 (CXCL8), RANTES (CCL5), and IP10 (CXCL10) via *Enzyme-Linked Immunosorbent Assay (ELISA). Cytokine IL6 was measured* via *a time-resolved fluorometry (TRF) detection system (DELFIA, Wallac, Turku, Finland)* [22, 30, 31], *and IL8, RANTES, and IP10 by colorimetric absorbance as per the manufacturer's instructions.*

3.7.1 Interleukin 6 ELISA (See Fig. 2a, b)

1. Collect supernatant from the basolateral compartment and washes from the apical surface of the differentiated nasal

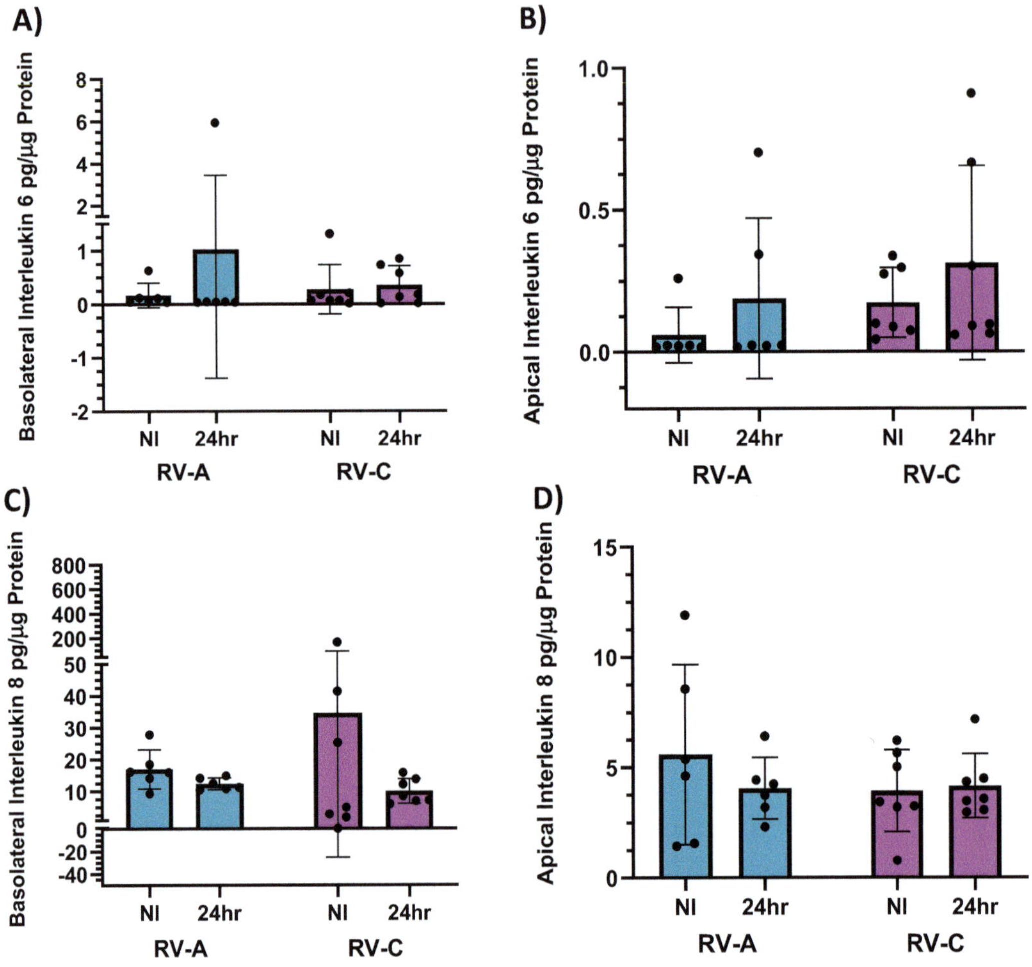

Fig. 2 (**a**) Basolateral levels of IL6 in non-infected NEC cultures (NI) and at 24 h post-infection with RV-A16 or RV-C15; (**b**) Apical levels of IL6 in non-infected NEC cultures and at 24 h post-infection with RV-A16 or RV-C15; (**c**) Basolateral levels of IL8 in non-infected NEC cultures and at 24 h post-infection with RV-A16 or RV-C15; (**d**) Apical levels of IL8 in non-infected NEC cultures (NI) and at 24 h post-infection with RV-A16 or RV-C15. Data points are representative of the assay

epithelial culture at the experimental designated timepoints and store at −80 °C until use.

2. Coat high-binding 96-well plates (NUNC Maxisorp, Thermo Fisher Scientific, Waltham, MA, USA) with 50 µL per well of monoclonal primary (capture) antibody (Clone: MQ2-13A5, catalogue# 554543, 0.5 mg/mL, BD Pharmingen, Sydney, NSW, Australia) diluted in coating buffer (1 plate: 2 µg/mL,) and cover with a plate sealer prior to incubating at 4 °C overnight.
3. Thaw blocking buffer at 4 °C overnight.

4. Thaw samples to room temperature. Nasal epithelial samples are typically not diluted for IL6 ELISA (neat). This can be optimized for specific samples.
5. Remove the coating buffer and add 300 μL of blocking buffer to each well on the 96-well plate and cover with a plate sealer prior to incubating on an orbital shaker for 1 h at room temperature.
6. To generate a linear standard curve, recombinant IL6 (catalogue# 550071, BD Pharmingen, Sydney, NSW, Australia) should be reconstituted and serially diluted (30,000, 10,000, 3000, 1000, 300, 100, 30, 10, 3, 1, 0.3, 0 (blank) pg/mL) in DELFIA Assay Buffer (DELFIA, Wallac, Turku, Finland).
7. Remove the blocking buffer and wash plates in 1× TRF Wash Buffer 5 times before blotting them dry.
8. Add 50 μL standards and samples to the plate as per the designated plate layout.
9. Cover the plates with plate sealers and incubate on an orbital shaker for 1 h at room temperature.
10. Biotinylated secondary antibody (catalogue# 554546, 0.5 mg/mL, BD Pharmingen, Sydney, NSW, Australia) should be diluted in DELFIA Assay Buffer (1 plate: 1 μg/mL) approximately 10 min prior to the end of primary antibody incubation.
11. Remove the standards and samples from the plate and wash with 1× TRF Wash Buffer 5 times before blotting them dry.
12. Add 50 μL of biotinylated secondary antibody to each well of the plate.
13. Cover the plates with plate sealers and incubate on an orbital shaker for 1 h at room temperature.
14. Europium-labelled Streptavidin Peroxidase (catalogue# 1244–360, Perkin-Elmer, Wallac, Turku, Finland) should be diluted in DELFIA Assay Buffer (1 plate: 1 μg/mL approximately 10 min prior to the end of biotinylated secondary antibody incubation.
15. Remove the biotinylated secondary antibody and wash plates in 1× TRF Wash Buffer 5 times before blotting them dry.
16. Add 50 μL of Europium-labelled Streptavidin Peroxidase to each well of the plate.
17. Cover the plates with plate sealers and incubate on an orbital shaker for 30 min at room temperature.
18. Move Enhancement Solution (DELFIA catalogue# 4001–0010, Perkin-Elmer, Wallac, Turku, Finland) from °C storage to room temperature away from light.

19. Remove the Europium-labelled Streptavidin Peroxidase wash plates in 1× TRF Wash Buffer 8 times before blotting them dry. Dry the underside of the plates thoroughly so as to avoid obscuring plate readings.
20. Add 50 μL of Enhancement Solution (DELFIA catalogue# 4001–0010, Perkin-Elmer, Wallac, Turku, Finland) to each well of the plate and do not cover with a plate sealer.
21. Incubate on an orbital shaker for 5 min at room temperature away from light.
22. Read time-resolved fluorescence on a plate reader.

3.7.2 BD OptEIA™ Interleukin 8 (CXCL8) ELISA (Catalogue# 555244, Becton Dickinson Biosciences, Franklin Lakes, NJ, USA) (See Fig. 2c, d)

1. Collect supernatant from the basolateral compartment and washes from the apical surface of the differentiated nasal epithelial culture at the experimental designated timepoints and store at −80 °C until use.
2. Coat half-area 96-well plates (COSTAR #3690, Corning, New York, NY, USA) with primary capture antibody diluted in coating buffer (working concentration as per the certificate of analysis) and cover with a plate sealer prior to incubating at 4 °C overnight.
3. Thaw samples to room temperature.
4. Remove the coating buffer and wash the plates in 1× IL8 Wash Buffer three times before blotting them dry.
5. Add 100 μL of Assay Diluent to each well of the plate, cover with a plate sealer, and incubate for 1 h at room temperature to block non-specific binding.
6. Optimization of sample dilutions is required for IL8 ELISA. For differentiated nasal epithelial cultures derived from acutely wheezing and non-wheezing children, the dilution factor was between 1:250 and 1:1000.
7. Dilute samples as required in Assay Diluent.
8. To generate a log standard curve, recombinant IL8 should be reconstituted and serially diluted in Assay Diluent (200, 100, 50, 25, 12.5, 6.3, 3.1, 0 (blank) pg/mL).
9. Remove the Assay Diluent and wash the plates in 1× IL8 Wash Buffer three times before blotting them dry.
10. Add 50 μL of standards and samples to designated wells in the plate before covering with a plate sealer and incubating for 2 h at room temperature.
11. Working Detector Antibody (Detection Antibody + SAv-HRP reagent, working concentration as per the Certificate of Analysis CoA) should be prepared 15 min prior to the end of the incubation.

12. Remove the standards and samples and wash the plates in 1× IL8 Wash Buffer five times before blotting them dry.
13. Add 50 μL of Working Detector Antibody to the designated wells in the plate, seal with a plate cover and incubate for 1 h at room temperature.
14. Remove the Working Detector Antibody and wash the plates in 1× IL8 Wash Buffer seven times for 30 s–1 min each before blotting them dry.
15. Add 50 μL 1-Step TMB ELISA Substrate Solution (Thermo Fisher Scientific, Waltham, MA, USA).
16. Incubate the plates without a plate sealer for 30 min at room temperature away from light.
17. Add 25 μL of Stop Solution (2 N H_2SO_4) to each well.
18. Read absorbance on a plate reader within 30 min of halting the reaction. Absorbance should be measured at a wavelength of 450 nm. It is recommended to simultaneously read at 570 nm and subtract this from the 450 nm reading for wavelength correction.

3.7.3 RANTES (CCL5) ELISA (R & D Systems, Minneapolis, MN, USA, Catalogue# DY278) (See Fig. 3a, b)

1. Collect supernatant from the basolateral compartment and washes from the apical surface of the differentiated nasal epithelial culture at the experimental designated timepoints and store at −80 until use.
2. Coat half-area 96-well plates (COSTAR #3690, Corning, New York, NY, USA) with 50 μL of Mouse Anti-Human primary capture antibody diluted in non-sterile 1× PBS to the working concentration as per the Certificate of Analysis (CoA) and cover with a plate sealer prior to incubating at room temperature overnight.
3. Thaw samples to room temperature. Nasal epithelial samples are typically not diluted for RANTES ELISA (neat). This can be optimized for specific samples.
4. Remove the Mouse Anti-Human primary capture antibody from the plates and wash the plates in 1× RANTES Wash Buffer three times before blotting them dry.
5. Add 150 μL of Reagent Diluent to each well of the plate, cover with a plate sealer, and incubate for 1 h at room temperature to block non-specific binding.
6. To generate a log standard curve, recombinant RANTES should be reconstituted as per the CoA and serially diluted in Assay Diluent (1000, 500, 250, 125, 62.5, 31.3, 15.6, 0 (blank) pg/mL).

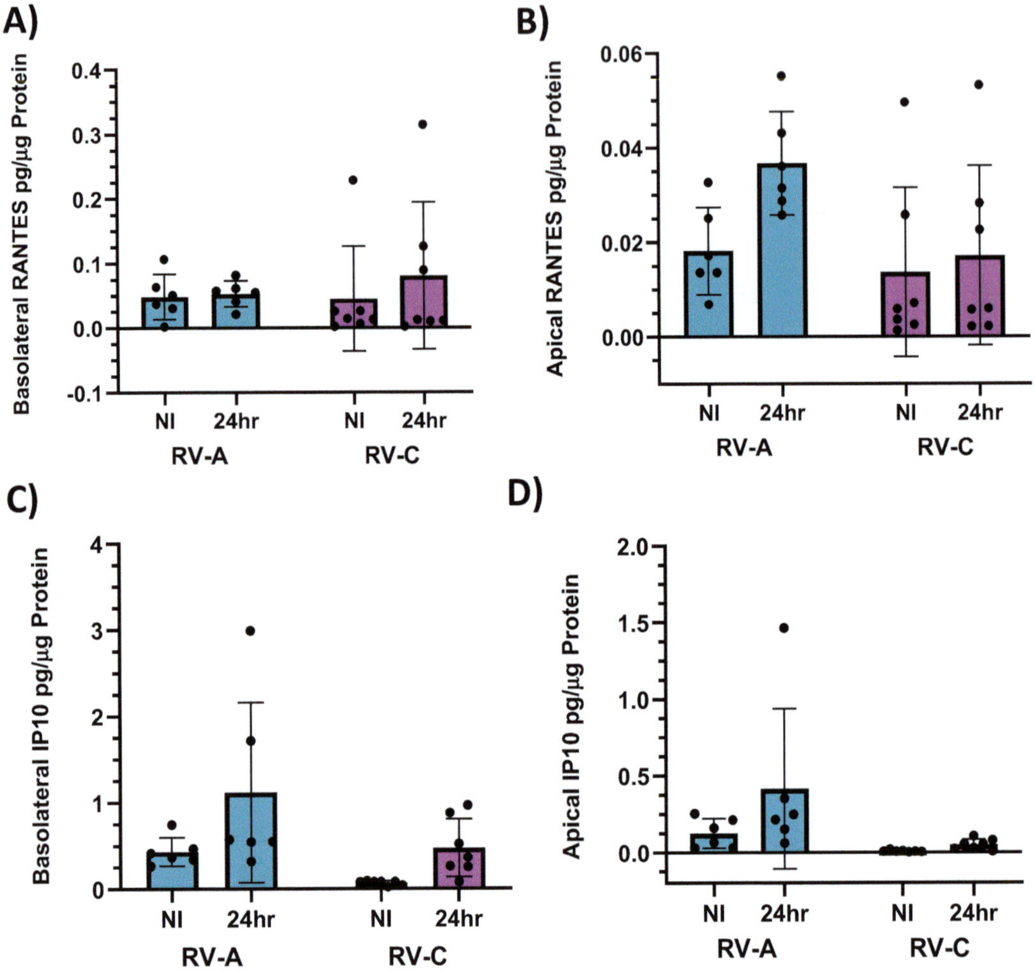

Fig. 3 (**a**) Basolateral levels of RANTES in non-infected NEC cultures (NI) and at 24 h post-infection with RV-A16 or RV-C15; (**b**) Apical levels of RANTES in non-infected NEC cultures and at 24 h post-infection with RV-A16 or RV-C15; (**c**) Basolateral levels of IP10 in non-infected NEC cultures and at 24 h post-infection with RV-A16 or RV-C15; (**d**) Apical levels of IP10 in non-infected NEC cultures (NI) and at 24 h post-infection with RV-A16 or RV-C15. Data points are representative of the assay

7. Remove the Reagent Diluent from the plates and wash the plates in 1× RANTES Wash Buffer three times before blotting them dry.
8. Add 50 μL of standards and samples to designated wells in the plate before covering with a plate sealer and incubating for 2 h at room temperature.
9. Dilute Biotinylated Goat Anti-Human RANTES Detection Antibody in Reagent Diluent as per the CoA.
10. Remove the standards and samples and wash the plates in 1× RANTES Wash Buffer three times before blotting them dry.

11. Add 50 μL of Biotinylated Goat Anti-Human RANTES Detection Antibody to the designated wells, cover with a plate sealer, and incubate for 2 h at room temperature.
12. Dilute Streptavidin-HRP in Reagent Diluent to the working dilution as per the CoA.
13. Remove the Biotinylated Goat Anti-Human RANTES Detection Antibody and wash the plates in 1× RANTES Wash Buffer three times before blotting them dry.
14. Add 50 μL of Streptavidin-HRP working dilution to the designated wells, cover with a plate sealer, and incubate for 20 min at room temperature away from light.
15. Remove the Streptavidin-HRP working dilution and wash the plates in 1× RANTES Wash Buffer three times before blotting them dry.
16. Add 50 μL 1-Step TMB ELISA Substrate Solution (Thermo Fisher Scientific, Waltham, MA, USA).
17. Incubate the plates without a plate sealer for 20 min at room temperature away from light.
18. Add 25 μL of Stop Solution (2 N H_2SO_4) to each well.
19. Read absorbance on a plate reader. Absorbance should be measured at a wavelength of 450 nm. It is recommended to simultaneously read at 540 nm or 570 nm and subtract this from the 450 nm reading for wavelength correction.

3.7.4 IP10 (CXCL10) ELISA (R & D Systems, Minneapolis, MN, USA) (See Fig. 3c, d)

1. Collect supernatant from the basolateral compartment and washes from the apical surface of the differentiated nasal epithelial culture at the experimental designated timepoints and store at −80 until use.
2. Coat half-area 96-well plates (COSTAR #3690, Corning, New York, NY, USA) with 50 μL of Mouse Anti-Human primary capture antibody diluted in non-sterile 1× PBS to the working concentration as per the Certificate of Analysis (CoA) and cover with a plate sealer prior to incubating at room temperature overnight.
3. Thaw samples to room temperature. Nasal epithelial samples are typically not diluted for RANTES ELISA (neat). This can be optimized for specific samples.
4. Remove the Mouse Anti-Human primary capture antibody from the plates and wash the plates in 1× IP10 Wash Buffer three times before blotting them dry.
5. Add 150 μL of Reagent Diluent to each well of the plate, cover with a plate sealer, and incubate for 1 h at room temperature to block non-specific binding.

6. To generate a log standard curve, recombinant IP10 should be reconstituted as per the CoA and serially diluted in Assay Diluent (2000, 1000, 500, 250, 125, 62.5, 31.3, 0 (blank) pg/mL).
7. Remove the Reagent Diluent from the plates and wash the plates in 1× IP10 Wash Buffer three times before blotting them dry.
8. Add 50 μL of standards and samples to designated wells in the plate before covering with a plate sealer and incubating for 2 h at room temperature.
9. Dilute Biotinylated Goat Anti-Human IP10 Detection Antibody in Reagent Diluent as per the CoA.
10. Remove the standards and samples and wash the plates in 1× IP10 Wash Buffer three times before blotting them dry.
11. Add 50 μL of Biotinylated Goat Anti-Human IP10 Detection Antibody to the designated wells, cover with a plate sealer, and incubate for 2 h at room temperature.
12. Dilute Streptavidin-HRP in Reagent Diluent to the working dilution as per the CoA.
13. Remove the Biotinylated Goat Anti-Human IP10 Detection Antibody and wash the plates in 1× IP10 Wash Buffer three times before blotting them dry.
14. Add 50 μL of Streptavidin-HRP working dilution to the designated wells, cover with a plate sealer, and incubate for 20 min at room temperature away from light.
15. Remove the Streptavidin-HRP working dilution and wash the plates in 1× IP10 Wash Buffer three times before blotting them dry.
16. Add 50 μL 1-Step TMB ELISA Substrate Solution (Thermo Fisher Scientific, Waltham, MA, USA).
17. Incubate the plates without a plate sealer for 20 min at room temperature away from light.
18. Add 25 μL of Stop Solution (2 N H_2SO_4) to each well.
19. Read absorbance on a plate reader. Absorbance should be measured at a wavelength of 450 nm. It is recommended to simultaneously read at 540 nm or 570 nm and subtract this from the 450 nm reading for wavelength correction.

3.7.5 Total Protein Quantification: Bicinchoninic Acid (BCA) Protein Assay (Pierce, Thermo Fisher Scientific, Waltham, MA, USA)

Total protein concentration is used to standardize the amount of specific cytokines, measured by ELISA, to the total protein concentration in each sample to achieve specific cytokine per 1 μg of total epithelial protein.

1. Submerge the differentiated nasal epithelial cell culture still attached to the insert membrane into Cell Extraction Buffer and pipette vigorously to lyse cells.
2. Dilute samples in 1:5 in non-sterile 1× PBS to a final volume of 25 μL/well.
3. To generate a linear standard curve, BSA should be diluted appropriately in non-sterile 1× PBS to achieve a range of standards from 20 to 2000 μg/mL. Include a standard that contains 0 μg/mL BSA as a blank for correction.
4. Add 25 μL of standards and samples in duplicate to designated wells on a 96-well plate (NUNC, Thermo Fisher Scientific, Waltham, MA, USA).
5. Add 50 parts Reagent A to 1 part Reagent B.
6. Add 25 μL of this mixture to the wells of the 96-well plate containing standards and samples.
7. Incubate the plate for 30 min at 37 °C and allow to cool.
8. Read absorbance at a wavelength of 562 nm.
9. Calculate μg/mL protein in each well and the total protein in each differentiated nasal epithelial culture by utilizing the linear standard curve.
10. Standardize ELISA data by calculating the amount of total target protein in each sample and dividing it by the total protein content of the cell culture to achieve the amount of target protein per 1 μg total protein.

3.8 Immunofluorescence and Confocal Microscopy: Cilia and Mucus (See Fig. 4a, b)

To detect the presence of cilia (beta-tubulin-IV) and mucin (MUC5AC), immunofluorescent (IF) staining and confocal microscope are used [32, 33].

3.8.1 Immunostaining

1. Submerge the differentiated nasal epithelial cell culture still attached to the insert membrane into fixative containing a 1:1 ratio of methanol and acetone for 10 min at −20 °C.
2. Remove fixative and replace with sterile 1× PBS prior to storing at 4 °C until use.
3. Permeabilize differentiated nasal epithelial cell cultures and block non-specific staining using one of the two methods below. Permeabilization method may need to be optimized for the designated target protein:
   - Transient permeabilization followed by blocking (used for protein targets where proteins on the edges of the cell may need to be preserved):

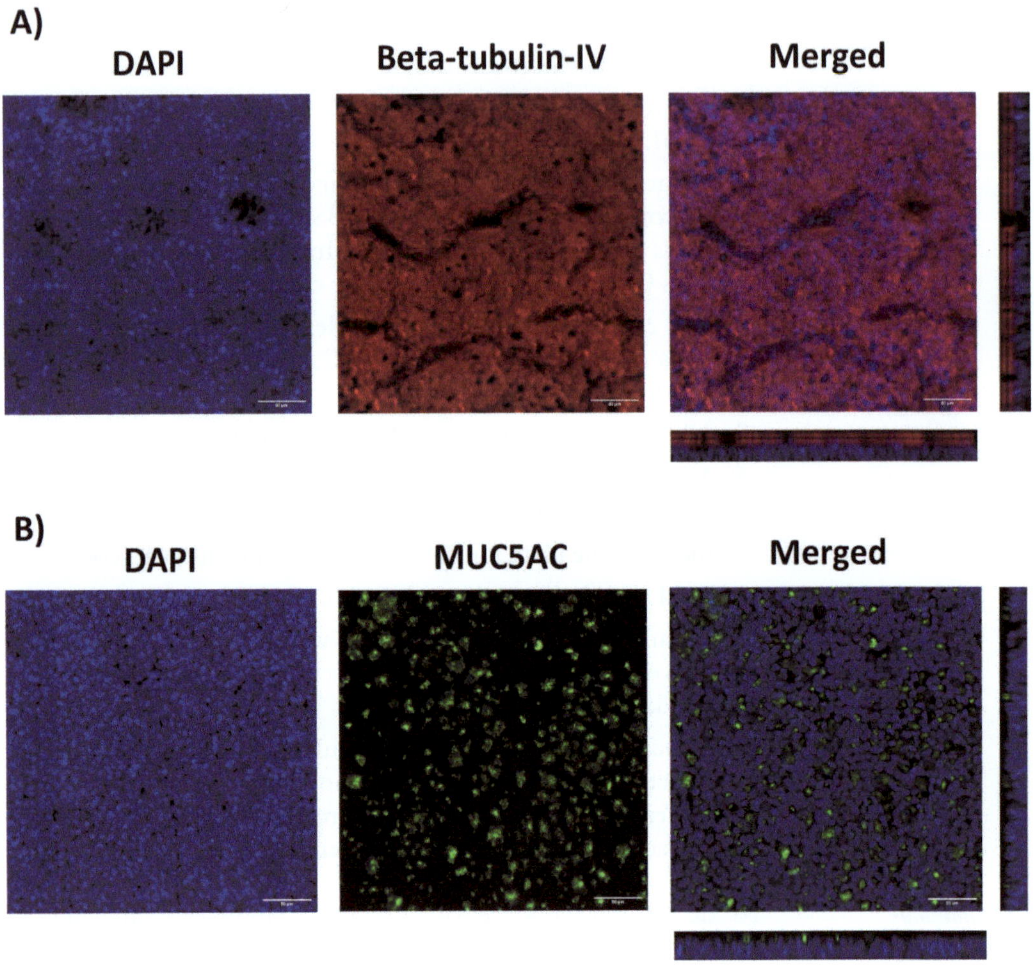

Fig. 4 (**a**) Immunostaining of Beta-tubulin-IV, indicative of cilia, in a fixed NEC culture with DAPI (nuclei) counterstaining. Image taken as a Z-Stack at 40× magnification; (**b**) Immunostaining of MUC5AC, indicative of mucus, in a fixed NEC culture with DAPI (nuclei) counterstaining. Image taken as a Z-Stack at 40× magnification. Images are representative of the method

1. Submerge the fixed culture in 0.1% (v/v) saponin (Sigma-Aldrich/Merck, St. Louis, MO, USA) in 1× TBS for 10 min at room temperature.
2. Remove saponin and wash the fixed culture in 1× TBS for 5 min at room temperature six times for a total of 30 min.
3. After removal of the last 1× TBS wash, submerge the fixed culture in IF Blocking Buffer for 30 min at room temperature.

- Permanent Permeabilization and concurrent Blocking:
  1. Submerge the fixed culture in Triton-×-100 Permeabilization and Blocking Solution for 30 min at room temperature.

Table 3
Primary antibodies for immunofluorescence

Primary antibody	Type	Dilution	Supplier
Beta-tubulin-IV	[ERP16776] rabbit polyclonal antibody	2.81 μg/mL	Cat #ab179509, 0.844 mg/mL AbCam, Cambridge, England
MUC5AC	(45 M1) Mouse monoclonal antibody	1 μg/mL	Cat #MA5-12178, 0.2 mg/mL Life technologies, Waltham, MA, USA

Table 4
Secondary antibodies for immunofluorescence

Secondary antibody	Fluorophore	Dilution	Supplier
Goat anti-mouse antibody	Alexa Fluor 488	5 μg/mL	Cat #A28175, 1 mg/mL Thermo fisher scientific, Waltham, MA, USA
Goat anti-rabbit antibody	Alexa Fluor 555	10 μg/mL	Cat #A21428, 2 mg/mL Thermo fisher scientific, Waltham, MA, USA

4. If using transient permeabilization, primary antibodies should be diluted in IF Blocking Buffer. If using permanent permeabilization, primary antibodies should be diluted in 1× TBS or Blocking Solution that does not contain Triton-×-100. Dilute primary antibodies (refer to Table 3 for primary antibodies) appropriately as per the recommended range in the supplier guidelines if available. For staining of beta-tubulin-IV and MUC5AC, the following dilutions have been used:
5. Incubate fixed cultures in the appropriate primary antibodies on a rocker or orbital shaker overnight at 4 °C [33].
6. Remove primary antibodies and wash fixed cultures in 1× TBS for 10 min at room temperature. Repeat this six times for a total of 1 h.
7. Dilute secondary antibodies (refer to Table 4 for secondary antibodies) in 1× TBS or Blocking Buffer appropriately as per the recommended range in the supplier guidelines if available. For staining of beta-tubulin-IV and MUC5AC, the following dilutions have been used:

8. After removing the last 1× TBS wash, incubate the fixed cultures in the appropriate secondary antibodies on a rocker or orbital shaker for 1 h at room temperature away from light.
9. Remove secondary antibodies and wash fixed cultures in 1× TBS for 10 min at room temperature. Repeat this five times for a total of 50 min.
10. For nuclei counterstaining, 4′,6-diamidino-2-phenylindole (DAPI, Sigma-Aldrich, St. Louis, MO, USA) should be diluted 1:10,000 in 1× TBS.
11. After removing the last 1× TBS wash, incubate the fixed cultures in DAPI on a rocker or orbital shaker for 5 min at room temperature.
12. Remove DAPI and wash fixed cultures on a rocker or orbital shaker in 1× TBS for 5 min at room temperature before removing.
13. Mount fixed cultures onto glass slides and cover with ProLong Diamond Anti-fade Mountant (Invitrogen, Waltham, MA, USA).
14. Add a #1.5 coverslip (source?) over the top of the fixed culture and mountant, being careful not to move the culture or trap air between the slide and coverslip. Seal the edges of the coverslip with nail polish.
15. Keep slides away from light and let the slides set until the nail polish is completely dry.

3.8.2 Acquisition of Z-Stack Images Through Confocal (Laser Scanning) Microscopy

1. Place the slide containing fixed culture into the appropriate stage on the confocal microscope (Nikon C2 Inverted + A1Si spectral detector, Nikon, Tokyo, Japan).
2. Select the objective (example: Nikon Plan Apo VC 40× NA dry immersion) and image resolution on the NIS-AR Elements software.
3. Set pinhole size (airy units, AU).
4. Make sure that imaging of individual laser channels is captured sequentially, not concurrently, to minimize bleed-through.
5. Optimize the laser power, gain, and offset for the brightest plane of the staining in the fixed culture. Optimize for each channel separately. Over- or under-saturation of pixels should be avoided and can be determined using the look-up table (LUT) function. The intensity histogram can also be used in the absence of LUT. Laser power should be kept low so as not to risk photobleaching.

6. To acquire a Z-Stack image, determine the focal plane for the top and bottom of the fixed culture as well as the appropriate step-size (μm).
7. Keep a record of all parameters for imaging the first fixed culture; these should be used to image all subsequent treatment groups (uninfected, RV-A16, RV-C15, timepoints).

Acknowledgements

Protocols pertaining to propagation through reverse genetics of clinical isolates of RV (RV-A16 and RV-C15 cloned from the nasopharyngeal aspirate of children), plasmids containing the full-length genomic cDNA copies of these viruses, and expert advice were kindly provided by Dr. Yury A. Bochkov and Professor James E. Gern (University of Wisconsin-Madison, WI, USA).

This work was funded by the Western Australian Child Health Research Fund and the National Health and Medical Research Council; RLW was supported by a Research Training Program Scholarship (The University of Western Australia and the Australian Government) and an Award for Research Excellence from the Stan Perron Charitable Foundation; TI was funded by a Future Health and Research Innovation Fund Innovation Fellowship, and a Stan Perron Charitable Foundation People Fellowship; IAL was funded by the National Health and Medical Research Council; AK was funded by a Rothwell Family Fellowship and the National Health and Medical Research Council.

The authors thank the participants and their families in the Western Australian Epithelial Research Program (WAERP) and the Mechanisms of Acute Viral Respiratory Infection in Children (MAVRIC) cohorts for their contribution to this study. We would also like to thank the contribution and assistance of all the respiratory fellows, anesthetists, nurses, and hospital staff at Perth Children's Hospital (previously Princess Margaret Hospital) and St John of God Hospital Subiaco. The members of WAERP are: Anthony Kicic, Stephen M. Stick, Elizabeth Kicic-Starcevich, Amy Greenly, Angela Fuery, Samuel T Montgomery, Luke W Garratt, Kevin Looi, Erika N Sutanto, Thomas Iosifidis, Kak-Ming Ling, Daniel Laucirica, Renee Ng, Jane Choi, Samantha McLean, Craig Schofield, Matthew Poh, Nicole C Shaw, Kelly M Martinovich, Rebecca L Watkinson, Katherine Landwehr, Denby Evans, Minda Amin, Rickie Fraser-Jones, Emma Catchpole, Mitchell Hedges, Andrew Vaitekenas, Joshua Iszatt, Reanne Ho, Rohan Flint, Sourav Shyam, Jack Canning, Danush Murali, Aaron Gomes, Shyan Vijayasekaran, George Sim, Mairead Heaney, Paul Swan, Ian Forsyth, Tobias Schoep, Alexander Larcombe, Monica Hunter, Kate McGee, Nyssa Millington, Francis J Lannigan, Ricardo Bergesio, Bernard Lee.

References

1. Bochkov YA, Watters K, Ashraf S, Griggs TF, Devries MK, Jackson DJ et al (2015) Cadherin-related family member 3, a childhood asthma susceptibility gene product, mediates rhinovirus C binding and replication. Proc Natl Acad Sci USA 112(17):5485–5490
2. Griggs TF, Bochkov YA, Basnet S, Pasic TR, Brockman-Schneider RA, Palmenberg AC et al (2017) Rhinovirus C targets ciliated airway epithelial cells. Respir Res 18(1):84
3. Vignola AM, Campbell AM, Chanez P, Bousquet J, Paul-Lacoste P, Michel FB et al (1993) HLA-DR and ICAM-1 expression on bronchial epithelial cells in asthma and chronic bronchitis. Am Rev Respir Dis 148(3): 689–694
4. Gosset P, Tillie-Leblond I, Janin A, Marquette CH, Copin MC, Wallaert B et al (1995) Expression of E-selectin, ICAM-1 and VCAM-1 on bronchial biopsies from allergic and non-allergic asthmatic patients. Int Arch Allergy Immunol 106(1):69–77
5. Knight DA, Holgate ST (2003) The airway epithelium: structural and functional properties in health and disease. Respirology 8(4): 432–446
6. Ruiz García S, Deprez M, Lebrigand K, Cavard A, Paquet A, Arguel MJ et al (2019) Novel dynamics of human mucociliary differentiation revealed by single-cell RNA sequencing of nasal epithelial cultures. Development 146(20)
7. Hartsock A, Nelson WJ (2008) Adherens and tight junctions: structure, function and connections to the actin cytoskeleton. Biochim Biophys Acta 1778(3):660–669
8. Sparrow MP, Omari TI, Mitchell HW (1995) The epithelial barrier and airway responsiveness. Can J Physiol Pharmacol 73(2):180–190
9. Watkinson RL, Looi K, Laing IA, Cianferoni A, Kicic A (2021) Viral induced effects on a vulnerable epithelium; lessons learned from paediatric asthma and eosinophilic oesophagitis. Front Immunol 12:773600
10. Lopez-Souza N, Favoreto S, Wong H, Ward T, Yagi S, Schnurr D et al (2009) In vitro susceptibility to rhinovirus infection is greater for bronchial than for nasal airway epithelial cells in human subjects. J Allergy Clin Immunol 123(6):1384–90.e2
11. Martinez FD, Wright AL, Taussig LM, Holberg CJ, Halonen M, Morgan WJ (1995) Asthma and wheezing in the first six years of life. The group health medical associates. N Engl J Med 332(3):133–138
12. Jackson DJ, Gangnon RE, Evans MD, Roberg KA, Anderson EL, Pappas TE et al (2008) Wheezing rhinovirus illnesses in early life predict asthma development in high-risk children. Am J Respir Crit Care Med 178(7):667–672
13. Rubner FJ, Jackson DJ, Evans MD, Gangnon RE, Tisler CJ, Pappas TE et al (2017) Early life rhinovirus wheezing, allergic sensitization, and asthma risk at adolescence. J Allergy Clin Immunol 139(2):501–507
14. Bizzintino J, Lee WM, Laing IA, Vang F, Pappas T, Zhang G et al (2011) Association between human rhinovirus C and severity of acute asthma in children. Eur Respir J 37(5): 1037–1042
15. Annamalay AA, Jroundi I, Bizzintino J, Khoo SK, Zhang G, Lehmann D et al (2017) Rhinovirus C is associated with wheezing and rhinovirus a is associated with pneumonia in hospitalized children in Morocco. J Med Virol 89(4):582–588
16. Cox DW, Khoo S-K, Zhang G, Lindsay K, Keil AD, Knight G et al (2018) Rhinovirus is the most common virus and rhinovirus-C is the most common species in paediatric intensive care respiratory admissions. Eur Respir J 52(2):1800207
17. Holgate ST (2011) The sentinel role of the airway epithelium in asthma pathogenesis. Immunol Rev 242(1):205–219
18. Veerati PC, Troy NM, Reid AT, Li NF, Nichol KS, Kaur P et al (2020) Airway epithelial cell immunity is delayed during rhinovirus infection in asthma and COPD. Front Immunol 11:974
19. Gagliardi TB, Goldstein ME, Song D, Gray KM, Jung JW, Ignacio MA et al (2022) Rhinovirus C replication is associated with the endoplasmic reticulum and triggers cytopathic effects in an in vitro model of human airway epithelium. PLoS Pathog 18(1):e1010159
20. Looi K, Buckley AG, Rigby PJ, Garratt LW, Iosifidis T, Zosky GR et al (2018) Effects of human rhinovirus on epithelial barrier integrity and function in children with asthma. Clin Exp Allergy 48(5):513–524
21. Looi K, Troy NM, Garratt LW, Iosifidis T, Bosco A, Buckley AG et al (2016) Effect of human rhinovirus infection on airway epithelium tight junction protein disassembly and

transepithelial permeability. Exp Lung Res 42(7):380–395

22. Kicic A, Stevens PT, Sutanto EN, Kicic-Starcevich E, Ling KM, Looi K et al (2016) Impaired airway epithelial cell responses from children with asthma to rhinoviral infection. Clin Exp Allergy 46(11):1441–1455
23. Iosifidis T, Sutanto EN, Buckley AG, Coleman L, Gill EE, Lee AH et al (2020) Aberrant cell migration contributes to defective airway epithelial repair in childhood wheeze. JCI Insight 5(7)
24. Ashraf S, Brockman-Schneider R, Bochkov YA, Pasic TR, Gern JE (2013) Biological characteristics and propagation of human rhinovirus-C in differentiated sinus epithelial cells. Virology 436(1):143–149
25. Ashraf S, Brockman-Schneider R, Gern JE (2015) Propagation of rhinovirus-C strains in human airway epithelial cells differentiated at air-liquid interface. Methods Mol Biol 1221: 63–70
26. Bochkov YA, Palmenberg AC, Lee WM, Rathe JA, Amineva SP, Sun X et al (2011) Molecular modeling, organ culture and reverse genetics for a newly identified human rhinovirus C. Nat Med 17(5):627–632
27. Riss T, Niles A, Moravec R, Karassina N, Vidugiriene J (2004) Cytotoxicity assays: in vitro methods to measure dead cells. In: Markossian S, Grossman A, Brimacombe K, Arkin M, Auld D, Austin C et al (eds) Assay guidance manual. Eli Lilly & Company and the National Center for Advancing Translational Sciences, Bethesda
28. Stutts MJ, Boucher RC, Bromberg PA, Gatzy JT (1981) Effects of ammonium and nitrate salts on lon transport across the excised canine trachea. Toxicol Appl Pharmacol 60(1): 91–105
29. He JQ, Sandford AJ, Wang IM, Stepaniants S, Knight DA, Kicic A et al (2008) Selection of housekeeping genes for real-time PCR in atopic human bronchial epithelial cells. Eur Respir J 32(3):755–762
30. Kicic A, Sutanto EN, Stevens PT, Knight DA, Stick SM (2006) Intrinsic biochemical and functional differences in bronchial epithelial cells of children with asthma. Am J Respir Crit Care Med 174(10):1110–1118
31. Taylor AL, Hale J, Hales BJ, Dunstan JA, Thomas WR, Prescott SL (2007) FOXP3 mRNA expression at 6 months of age is higher in infants who develop atopic dermatitis, but is not affected by giving probiotics from birth. Pediatr Allergy Immunol 18(1):10–19
32. Martinovich KM, Iosifidis T, Buckley AG, Looi K, Ling KM, Sutanto EN et al (2017) Conditionally reprogrammed primary airway epithelial cells maintain morphology, lineage and disease specific functional characteristics. Sci Rep 7(1):17971
33. Buckley AG, Looi K, Iosifidis T, Ling KM, Sutanto EN, Martinovich KM et al (2018) Visualisation of multiple tight junctional complexes in human airway epithelial cells. Biol Proced Online 20:3

Chapter 11

In Vivo Model to Assess the Nasal Infection by Minor Group Rhinovirus

Umadevi Sajjan

Abstract

Rhinovirus primarily infects humans via nasal epithelial cells and is spread through the inhalation of shed progeny virus via micro-droplets containing the virus. A handful of studies have investigated the nasal mucosal responses to rhinovirus in experimentally infected healthy volunteers. There are also studies that have investigated the effect of antiviral drugs in reducing symptoms induced by rhinovirus infection. It is extremely expensive to test the antiviral drugs in human volunteers, and therefore having preclinical in vivo models is necessary to confirm the antiviral effect of the drugs prior to conducting clinical trials. The existing in vivo models for RV infection are focused on lung inflammation, which may be relevant to patients with chronic lung diseases, in whom rhinovirus causes lower respiratory tract infections. In this chapter, we describe a mouse model of rhinovirus infection, which shows self-limiting inflammation of the sinonasal mucosa.

Key words Interferon, Tight junctions, Mucus secretion, Inflammation

1 Introduction

Rhinovirus (RV) primarily infects the upper respiratory epithelium, frequently causing common colds in healthy subjects but more severe respiratory symptoms in patients with chronic lung diseases. To understand the mechanisms by which RV causes respiratory symptoms, various model systems have been used, including experimental rhinovirus infection in normal subjects, patients with asthma, and chronic obstructive pulmonary disease COPD) [1–4]. Normal healthy subjects showed upper respiratory symptoms that resolved within 7 days. However, patients with asthma and COPD showed increased upper respiratory symptoms, eventually developing lower respiratory symptoms. This is thought to be due to increased viral shedding in the nose and inhalation of the virus into the lungs [1]. In vivo models mimicking human infection are

Umadevi Sajjan (ed.), *Rhinovirus: Methods and Protocols*, Methods in Molecular Biology, vol. 2903,
https://doi.org/10.1007/978-1-0716-4410-2_11,

needed to understand the spread of the virus and the mechanisms underlying the severe disease caused by RV.

The experimental RV infection model has also been used to examine the efficacy of antiviral drugs in reducing the symptoms of the common cold and exacerbations in patients with asthma [5]. But so far, none of the drugs that were tested are on the market are effective in treating rhinovirus-related illnesses. The drug efficacy depends on the absorbance, rate of clearance of the drug, and availability of the drug in its active form at the site of infection. These parameters can be tested by using an appropriate in vivo model of infection. In this chapter, we describe an intranasal RV1B infection model that shows inflammation of the sinus mucosa and dissociation of E-cadherin in the nasal epithelium.

2 Materials

1. Six to eight weeks old C57BL/6 mice. The study must be approved by the Institutional Animal Care and User Committee.
2. Purified high-titer RV1B virus.
3. Endotoxin-free PBS.
4. TRIZOL.
5. Direct-zol RNA isolation kit (Zymo Research).
6. cDNA synthesis kit.
7. TaqMan probe-based assays and TaqMan qPCR reagents.
8. Rhinovirus-specific probe and primers for detection of virus.
9. One-step qPCR kit.
10. Plasmid containing a fragment of rhinovirus genome corresponding to PCR product.
11. Real-time PCR machine, Quantstudio 5 PCR machine, or similar.
12. 10% neutral-buffered formalin.
13. StatLab™ RapidCal Immuno Decalcifier.
14. Rabbit monoclonal antibody to E-cadherin (Cell signaling, Cat # 3195).
15. Antirabbit IgG coupled with AF 488.
16. Normal goat IgG.
17. Fluorescent mounting medium (Agilient DAKO cat# S3023).
18. DAPI (4′,6-diamidino-2-phenylindole) (Cell signaling, Cat# 4083). Prepare 1 mg/mL DAPI in DMSO and store in aliquots.

19. Coplin Jars.
20. Microwave.
21. PAP Pen for Immunostaining (Millipore Sigma Cat# Z377821).
22. Humidified chamber for staining slides (Millipore/Sigma cat # Z670146). The humidified chamber can also be created with a shallow plastic box with a lid as follows. Place a wet paper towel in a shallow plastic dish. Place serological pipettes horizontally and close the lid to create a humidified chamber. The slides must be on the serological pipettes to avoid the water from the wet paper towels mixing with antibodies.
23. 10 mM citric acid buffer pH 6.0.
24. Isoflurane inhalation anesthesia machine.
25. Angio catheter 22 gauge.
26. Light microscope with color camera.
27. Fluorescence microscope with CCD camera.

3 Methods

3.1 Preparation for RV1B Virus

RV1B binds to low-density lipoprotein receptor family members and infects mouse airway epithelial cells in vitro and mouse airways in vivo [6]. This serotype has been used extensively to determine the lower respiratory responses in mouse models of asthma and COPD [7–12]. The virus for these studies can be propagated in H1HeLa cells maintained in serum-free media after infection. The virus should be purified by ultrafiltration to 3×10^8 to 1×10^9 pfu/mL using endotoxin-free PBS for dialysis (*see* **Note 1**). The method for propagation of the virus is described in Chapter 2.

3.2 Intranasal Infection of Mice with Rhinovirus

1. Anesthetize 6–8-week-old mice in an isoflurane inhalation anesthesia machine with 20% isoflurane and 80% oxygen until they are completely anesthetized, which takes approximately 5–10 min (*see* **Note 2**).
2. Remove the mouse from the anesthesia machine and hold it in the palm at a 45-degree angle with the back of the mouse lying on the palm (*see* Fig. 1).
3. With a sterile filter pipette tip, apply 20 μL of virus (5×10^6 pfu) diluted in endotoxin-free PBS dropwise on the nares of the mice. Hold the mouse in the same position until they aspirate all the liquid.
4. For control mice, instill 20 μL of sham prepared from uninfected H1HeLa cell cultures and purified similarly to RV.

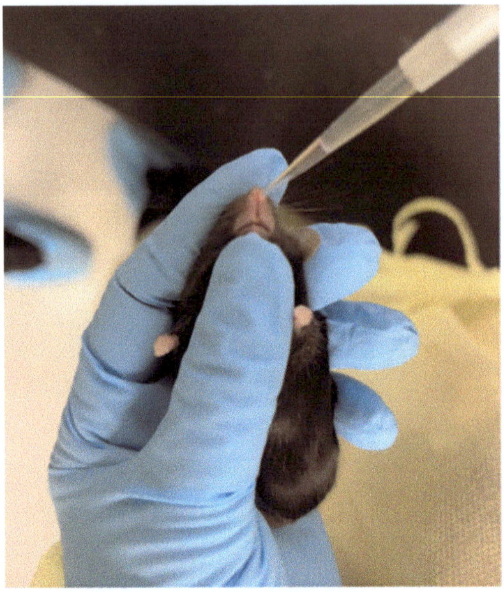

Fig. 1 Intranasal infection of mice. Hold the mouse at a 45-degree angle with the mouth closed. Instill the virus dropwise into the nares and wait until each drop is aspirated before instilling another drop to prevent the loss of infection volume

3.3 Lysis of Sinonasal Cells with TRIZOL for RNA Extraction

1. Sacrifice mice by asphyxiation at days 1, 3, 4, and 7 post-infection.
2. Make a small incision on the ventral side below the neck of the mice (*see* Fig. 2).
3. Insert an Angio catheter through the trachea towards the nose.
4. Slowly inject 0.5 mL of Trizol into the Angio catheter (*see* **Note 3**).
5. Collect the Trizol lysate of the sinus and nasal cavities from the nose.
6. Extract the RNA following the manufacturer's instructions.

3.4 Quantification of Rhinovirus in the Nasal Mucosa by qPCR

1. RV cDNA plasmid to create a standard curve. Prepare dilutions of RV cDNA plasmid from 10 to 1×10^9 copies per 5 μL.
2. The rhinovirus can be quantified by one-step qPCR using the following primers and probe:

   Sense primer: 5′-GTG AAG AGC CSC RTG TGC T-3′.

   Antisense primer: e 5′-GCT SCA GGG TTA AGG TTA GCC-3′.

   Probe: 5′-FAM-TGA GTC CTC CGG CCC CTG AAT G-TAMRA-3′

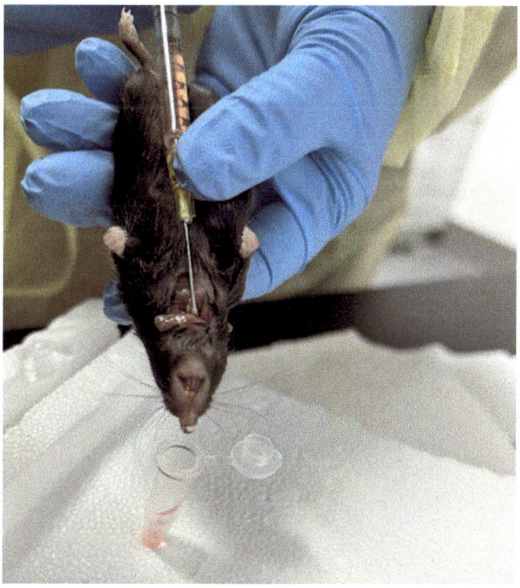

Fig. 2 Make a small incision below the neck area, and tease the muscles and the connective tissue to expose the trachea. Be careful not to damage the blood vessels. Insert a needle or Angio catheter and hold the mouse in the inverted position and slowly inject the TRIZOL and collect the sinonasal lysate from the nose

3. Set up of PCR reaction mix:

2× PCR master mix	10 μL
50 nM sense primer	2 μL
300 nM antisense primer	2 μL
175 nM probe	2 μL
RNA	0.2 μg in 5 μL
Water to	20 μL

4. Make up sufficient PCR master mix without adding RNA. Aliquot into designated wells in the 96-well PCR plate. Add RNA sample or cDNA. Seal the PCR plate with an optical adhesive cover.
5. Run the PCR Quantstudio 5 PCR machine using the program for quantitation with a standard curve.
6. Define the standards with the amount of viral RNA copy number.
7. Define the samples.
8. Set up the run program following the manufacturer's instructions (from where the qPCR reagents are purchased), except for the annealing temperature, which is set at 58 ° C.

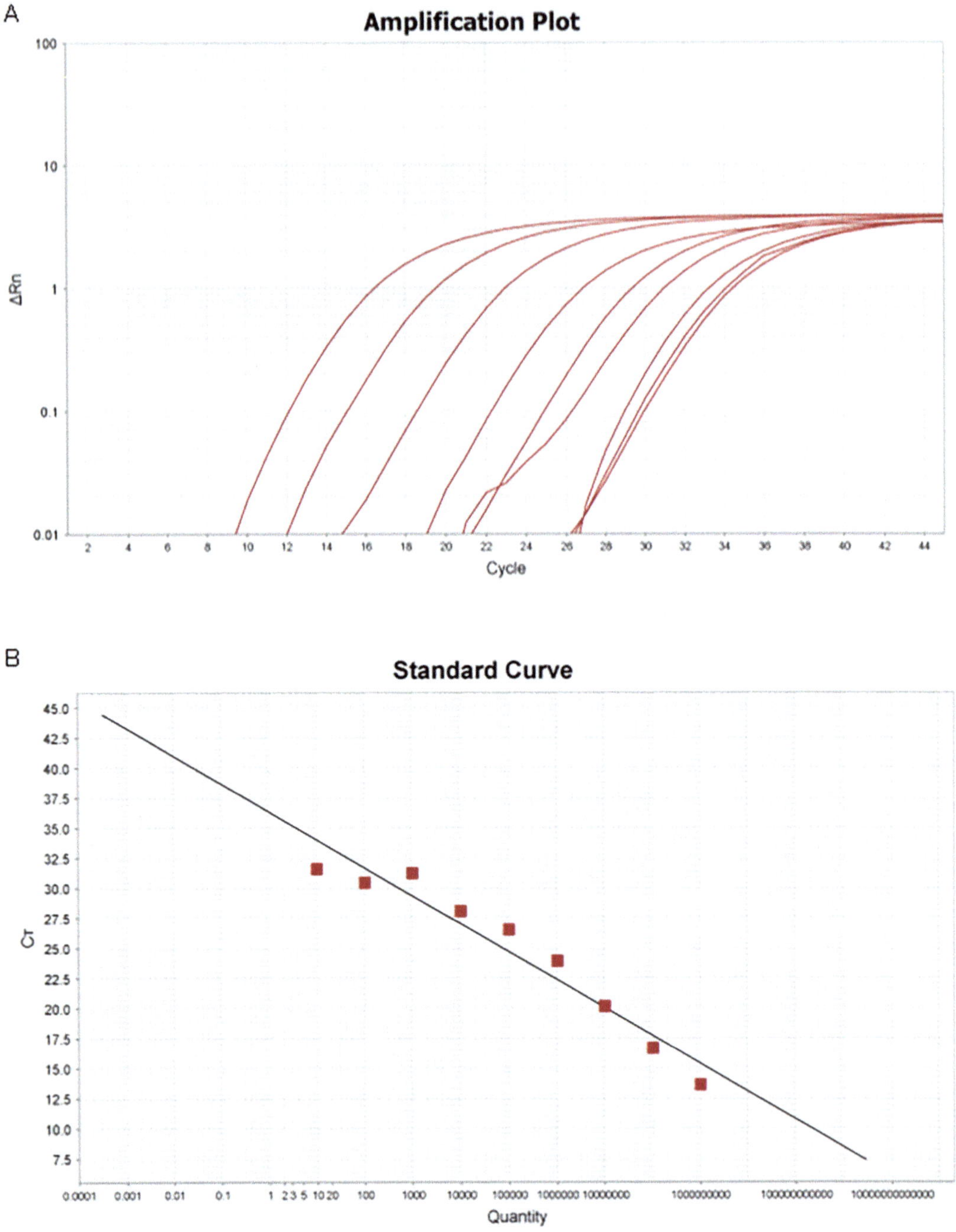

Fig. 3 PCR amplification of virus cDNA standards for quantification of RV. When setting up the qPCR machine, chose the quantitative PCR method with a standard curve. Define the standards and the negative control and then choose the probe. Run the qPCR and analyze the results. (**a**). Set the view to visualize amplification curves to confirm the specificity. The curves in the figure represent amplification curves from different amounts of RV cDNA. (**b**). The standard curve generated from the qPCR machine. The higher the cDNA, lower the Ct values therefore the curve show negative correlation. One can also generate the standard curve after analysis by using other software, such as GraphPad or Excel, which can be used for the integration of Ct values from the unknowns (*see* Fig. 4)

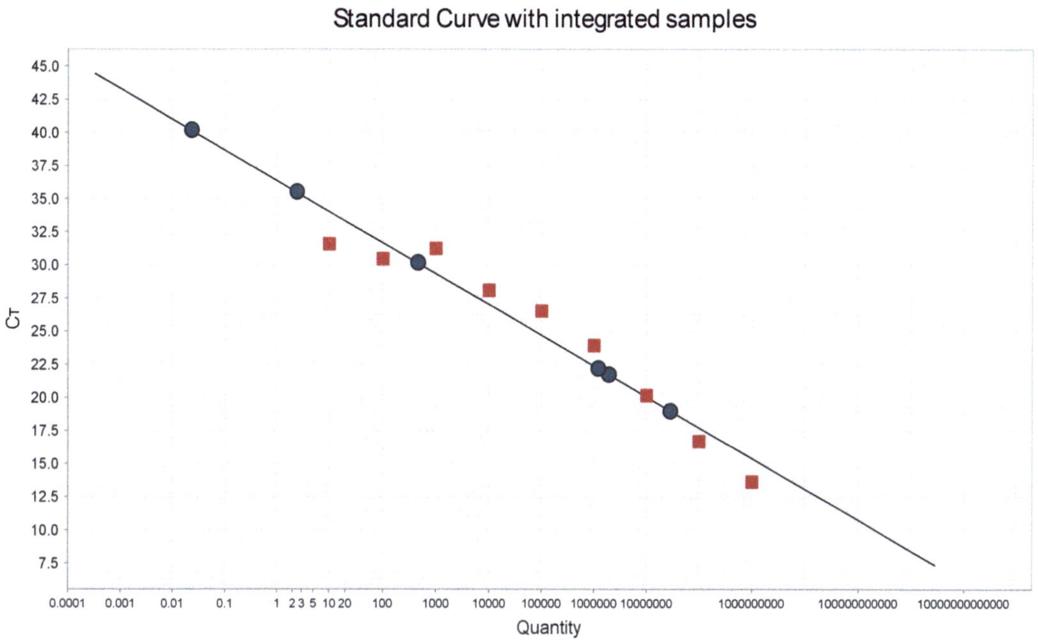

Fig. 4 qPCR for determination of RV RNA copy number. Conduct the qPCR by using the method of quantification with a standard curve. Always run the known copy number of viral RNA along with the samples. Generate the standard curve, and the machine will automatically integrate the samples into the standard curve and calculate the viral copy number in the sample, which can be exported by using the export tab (red squares, known copy number of viral RNA, and dark blue circles, samples integrated into the standard curve)

9. After analysis, create the standard curve with the known copy number of viral RNA. Amplification curves for standards are shown in Fig. 3a, and the standard curve is generated in Fig. 3b.
10. Calculate the amount of viral RNA by integrating the Ct values of samples into the standard curve (Fig. 4). Express the results as the number of viral RNA copies per μg of total RNA (*see* **Note 4**).

3.5 Determination of mRNA Expression of Cytokines and Antiviral Interferons

1. Convert the RNA to cDNA using a cDNA synthesis kit following the manufacturer's instructions.
2. Using gene-specific TaqMan assays, determine the expression of relevant inflammatory and interferon genes by real-time PCR and normalize the mRNA expression to the housekeeping gene β-actin.
3. We usually determine the expression of CXCL-1, CXCL-2, CXCL-10, TNF-α, IL-6, IFN-β, and IFN-λ1/2. All these genes are stimulated by RV1B in mice.

3.6 Assessment of Histology of the Nose

1. With a sharp razor blade or scalpel, cut the snout just below the eyes.
2. Remove the skin and remove the lower jaw.
3. Fix the upper jaw containing sinus tissue in 10% neutral-buffered formalin for at least 24 h at 4 ° C.
4. Place the tissue in 20 volumes of StatLab™ RapidCal Immuno Decalcifier.
5. Incubate for 12–16 h at room temperature.
6. Rinse the tissue well in water.
7. Incubate the tissue in 50% ethanol with two changes at 30 min intervals.
8. Incubate the tissue in 70% ethanol with two changes at 30 min intervals.
9. Process the tissue in the tissue processer using the following program in Table 1.
10. Embed the tissue in the paraffin.
11. Cut 5 μ thick sections and stain with hematoxylin and eosin (H & E) or periodic acid Schiff's reagent to detect goblet cells.
12. H & E-stained sections from mice infected with RV1B show mucus secretion and mild inflammation (*see* Fig. 5).

Table 1
Tissue processer

Step	Reagent (with % concentration)	Temp (°C)	Vacuum	Immersion Hours: minutes	Drain time Minutes: seconds
1	70% ethanol	A	Y	**1:00**	0:30
2	80% ethanol	A	Y	**1:00**	1:00
3	95% ethanol	A	Y	**1:00**	1:00
4	95% ethanol	A	Y	**1:00**	1:00
5	100% ethanol	A	Y	**1:00**	1:00
6	100% ethanol	A	Y	**1:00**	1:00
7	100% ethanol	A	Y	**1:00**	2:00
8	Xylenes	A	Y	**1:00**	1:00
9	Xylenes	A	Y	**1:00**	1:00
10	Xylenes	A	Y	**1:00**	2:00
11	Paraffin	60	Y	**1:00**	2:00
12	Paraffin	60	Y	**1:00**	2:00
13	Paraffin	60	Y	**1:00**	2:00
			Program duration: approximately 14.25 hrs.		

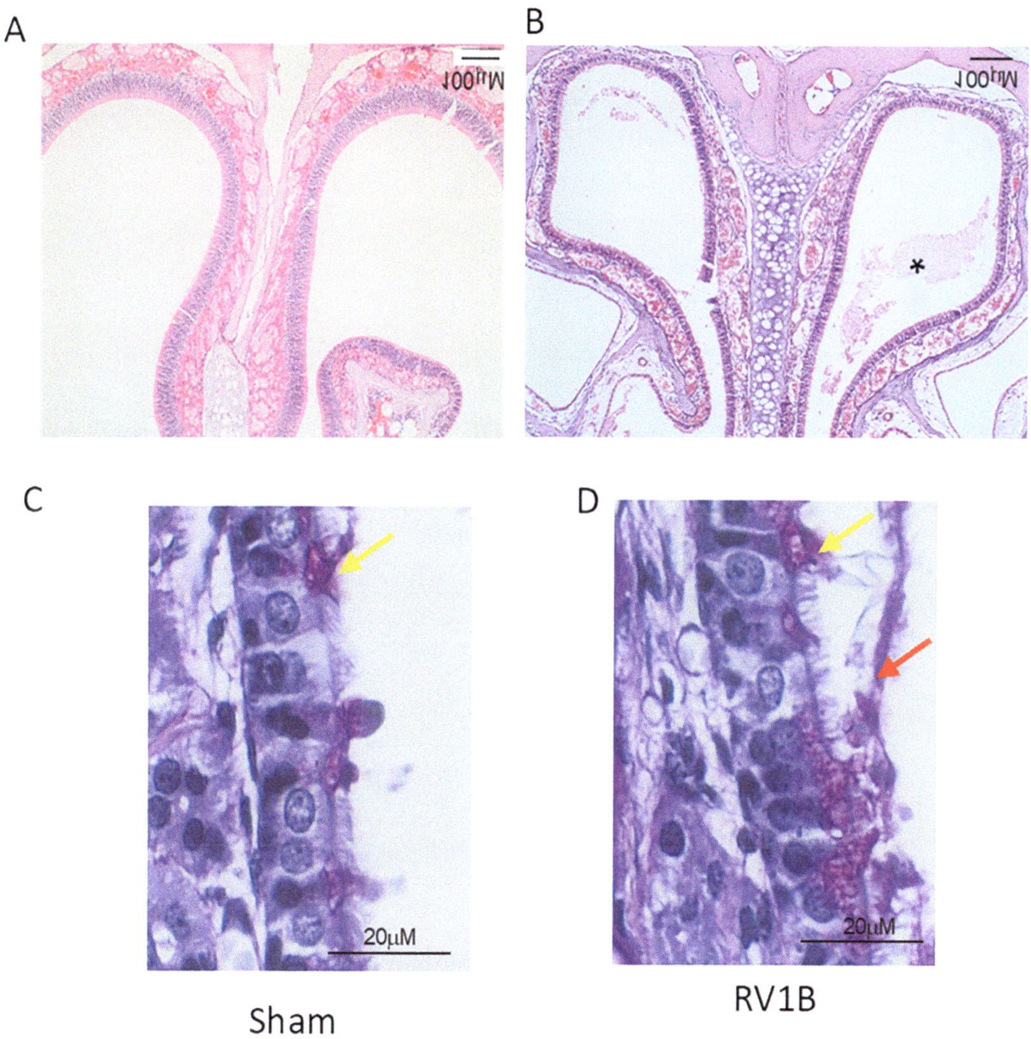

Fig. 5 Mice were infected with sham or RV1B and sacrificed on Day 4, and the mouse nose was processed for histology. (**a** and **b**). H and E-stained sections showing the sinus cavity lined with the epithelium. Asterisk in panel B represents mucus accumulation with some inflammatory cells. (**c** and **d**). Pas-stained sections showing goblet cells (yellow arrow) and secreted mucus (red arrow)

3.7 Expression of E-Cadherin in the Nasal Epithelium by Immunofluorcsccncc

Previously, we have shown that RV infection disrupts intercellular junctions in the mouse airway epithelium [13]. This can be visualized by determining the localization of one of the proteins of tight or adherence junctions. The following describes the method used for the localization of E-cadherin, an adherence junction protein, by immunofluorescence microscopy.

1. Cut 5 μ thick sections.
2. Hydrate the sections in xylene followed by graded alcohol and water as follows:
   1. Xylene 3 × 5′.
   2. 100% alcohol 2 × 5′
   3. 90% alcohol 2 × 5′
   4. 80% alcohol 2 × 5′
   5. 60% alcohol 2 × 5′
   6. 40% alcohol 2 × 5′
   7. Water 3 × 5′.
3. Boil the citric acid buffer in a Coplin jar in the microwave. Immerse the slides in boiling citric acid buffer and continue to boil for 10 min at a low power level. This step is used for unmasking antigenic sites.
4. Let the Coplin jar, along with the buffer and slides, cool to room temperature.
5. Wash slides in water 3 × 10′.
6. Wash slides in PBS 3 × 10′.
7. Draw a hydrophobic ring around the sections with a PAP pen. This is important to hold the antibody or blocking solutions on the sections.
8. Add 200 μL of 5% normal goat IgG (blocking buffer) on tissue sections and incubate for a minimum of 2 h in a humidified chamber.
9. Remove the blocking buffer by flicking the slide.
10. Add 100–200 μL of 1:500 diluted E-cadherin antibody and incubate overnight at 4 ° C in a humidified chamber.
11. Wash the slide in PBS 3 × 10′ to remove unbound antibody.
12. Add 100–200 μL of 1:100 diluted antirabbit IgG conjugated with AF 888 and incubate at room temperature for 1 h.
13. Wash the slide in PBS 3 × 10′ to remove the unbound second antibody.
14. Add DAPI (100 ng/mL) diluted in PBS to sections and incubate for 15 min at room temperature in a humidified chamber to counterstain the nuclei.
15. Mount the sections using fluorescent mounting medium.
16. Representative images of mouse nasal sections from sham and RV infected animals showing localization is presented in Fig. 6. This figure shows intermittent dissociation of E-cadherin from the intercellular junctions of nasal epithelium.

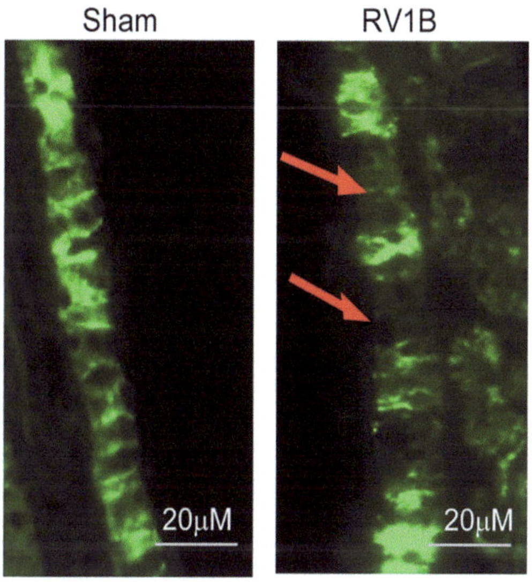

Fig. 6 Immunolocalization of E-cadherin. Five-micron-thick sections were deparaffinized, hydrated, and treated with citric acid to unmask the antigenic sites. The sections were blocked and incubated with primary antibody overnight at 4 °C. After washing unbound antibody, the bound antibody was detected by a second antibody conjugated to AF 488 and visualized under a fluorescence microscope

This model also shows an increase in the expression of several cytokines and antiviral interferons. The most robust responses are expressions of TNF-α, CXCL-10, and type I and type III interferons. This model also shows distinct histological changes with increased mucus secretion. Therefore, this model can be used to test the efficacy of antiviral drugs. This model can also be adapted to investigate the RV-induced pathogenesis in the nares of mouse models of asthma and COPD and the spread of the virus to the lower respiratory tract.

4 Notes

1. The use of endotoxin-free PBS during ultrafiltration, which combines dialysis and concentration of the virus or sham, is critical. The presence of endotoxin even in small amounts will stimulate inflammation even in sham-infected animals, which is indistinguishable from inflammation caused by RV.
2. Mice anesthetized with isoflurane inhalation will wake up within 1 or 2 min. Therefore, it is extremely important to complete the instillation of the virus within that period. If the mice are anesthetized too deeply, the mice may die during the infection.

3. For collecting TRIZOL lysates of sinunasal mucosa, hold the mouse head down so that the drops of TRIZOL coming from the nares can be collected in a tube. Do not use more than 0.5 mL TRIZOL. The TRIZOL will enter the mouth and will contaminate sinonasal RNA.
4. In parallel, one can also amplify the housekeeping gene using the same amount of RNA, and vRNA copies can then be expressed in relation to copies of the housekeeping gene.

References

1. Adura PT, Reed E, Macintyre J, Del Rosario A, Roberts J, Pestridge R, Beegan R, Boxall CB, Xiao C, Kebadze T, Aniscenko J, Cornelius V, Gern JE, Monk PD, Johnston SL, Djukanovic R (2014) Experimental rhinovirus 16 infection in moderate asthmatics on inhaled corticosteroids. Eur Respir J 43:1186–1189
2. Mallia P, Message SD, Gielen V, Contoli M, Gray K, Kebadze T, Aniscenko J, Laza-Stanca-V, Edwards MR, Slater L, Papi A, Stanciu LA, Kon OM, Johnson M, Johnston SL (2011) Experimental rhinovirus infection as a human model of chronic obstructive pulmonary disease exacerbation. Am J Respir Crit Care Med 183:734–742
3. Mallia P, Message SD, Kebadze T, Parker HL, Kon OM, Johnston SL (2006) An experimental model of rhinovirus induced chronic obstructive pulmonary disease exacerbations: a pilot study. Respir Res 7:116
4. Message SD, Laza-Stanca V, Mallia P, Parker HL, Zhu J, Kebadze T, Contoli M, Sanderson G, Kon OM, Papi A, Jeffery PK, Stanciu LA, Johnston SL (2008) Rhinovirus-induced lower respiratory illness is increased in asthma and related to virus load and Th1/2 cytokine and IL-10 production. Proc Natl Acad Sci USA 105:13562–13567
5. Coultas JA, Cafferkey J, Mallia P, Johnston SL (2021) Experimental antiviral therapeutic studies for human rhinovirus infections. J Exp Pharmacol 13:645–659
6. Newcomb DC, Sajjan US, Nagarkar DR, Wang Q, Nanua S, Zhou Y, McHenry CL, Hennrick KT, Tsai WC, Bentley JK, Lukacs NW, Johnston SL, Hershenson MB (2008) Human rhinovirus 1B exposure induces phosphatidylinositol 3-kinase-dependent airway inflammation in mice. Am J Respir Crit Care Med 177:1111–1121
7. Nagarkar DR, Bowman ER, Schneider D, Wang Q, Shim J, Zhao Y, Linn MJ, McHenry CL, Gosangi B, Bentley JK, Tsai WC, Sajjan US, Lukacs NW, Hershenson MB (2010) Rhinovirus infection of allergen-sensitized and -challenged mice induces eotaxin release from functionally polarized macrophages. J Immunol 185:2525–2535
8. Sajjan U, Ganesan S, Comstock AT, Shim J, Wang Q, Nagarkar DR, Zhao Y, Goldsmith AM, Sonstein J, Linn MJ, Curtis JL, Hershenson MB (2009) Elastase- and LPS-exposed mice display altered responses to rhinovirus infection. Am J Physiol Lung Cell Mol Physiol 297:L931–L944
9. Rajput C, Han M, Ishikawa T, Lei J, Jazaeri S, Bentley JK, Hershenson MB (2020) Early-life heterologous rhinovirus infections induce an exaggerated asthma-like phenotype. J Allergy Clin Immunol 146:571–582
10. Han M, Ishikawa T, Bermick JR, Rajput C, Lei J, Goldsmith AM, Jarman CR, Lee J, Bentley JK, Hershenson MB (2020) IL-1beta prevents ILC2 expansion, type 2 cytokine secretion, and mucus metaplasia in response to early-life rhinovirus infection in mice. Allergy 75:2005–2019
11. Gimenes JA Jr, Srivastava V, ReddyVari H, Kotnala S, Mishra R, Farazuddin M, Li W, Sajjan US (2019) Rhinovirus-induces progression of lung disease in a mouse model of COPD via IL-33/ST2 signaling axis. Clin Sci (Lond) 133: 983–996
12. Gimenes-Junior J, Owuar N, Vari HR, Li W, Xander N, Kotnala S, Sajjan US (2019) FOXO3a regulates rhinovirus-induced innate immune responses in airway epithelial cells. Sci Rep 9:18180
13. Sajjan U, Wang Q, Zhao Y, Gruenert DC, Hershenson MB (2008) Rhinovirus disrupts the barrier function of polarized airway epithelial cells. Am J Respir Crit Care Med 178: 1271–1281

Chapter 12

Identification and Analysis of Type 2 Innate Lymphoid Cells in Rhinovirus-Infected Mouse Model of Asthma

Charu Rajput

Abstract

Early-life respiratory tract infections by rhinovirus (RV) are considered risk factors for asthma development. Previous studies have shown that RV infection of six-day-old BALB/c mice, but not mature mice, induces an asthma-like phenotype, including mucous metaplasia and airway hyperresponsiveness, which is associated with the expansion of type 2 innate lymphoid cells (ILC2s). This chapter describes the isolation and analysis of ILC2s from RV-infected neonatal mouse lungs by flow cytometry, in vitro culture and adoptive transfer.

Key words Rhinovirus, ILC2s, in vitro culture, Immunofluorescence, Adoptive transfer, Flow cytometry

1 Introduction

The development of asthma results from various factors such as genetic predisposition, immune dysfunction and environmental exposures in early infancy. Epidemiologic studies in high-risk infants indicate that early-life respiratory viral infection, particularly with rhinovirus (RV), is a major predisposing factor for asthma development [1–4]. Because the airway epithelium is a major target of respiratory viral infection, the epithelium-derived cytokines IL-25, IL-33, and TSLP and their downstream cellular targets are uniquely positioned to play a role in viral-induced chronic airway disease. Previously, it has been shown that RV infection of six-day-old, but not mature mice, induces mucous metaplasia and airway hyperresponsiveness, which is accompanied by airway epithelial cell IL-25, IL-33 and TSLP production, and expansion of IL-13-producing type 2 innate lymphoid cells (ILC2s) [5].

ILC2s are morphologically similar to lymphocytes but do not express T- or B-cell receptors or surface markers associated with other immune cell lineages. ILC2s express cluster of differentiation

Umadevi Sajjan (ed.), *Rhinovirus: Methods and Protocols*, Methods in Molecular Biology, vol. 2903,
https://doi.org/10.1007/978-1-0716-4410-2_12,

90 (CD90)/Thyl, CD25 (IL-2Rα) and CD127 (IL-7Rα), and their development is dependent on the common γ-chain (γc or CD132), IL-7, Notch, DNA-binding protein inhibitor 2 (Id2), GATA3, and retinoic acid receptor-related orphan receptor-α [6–8].

We present here methods for flow cytometry and sorting of ILC2s from RV-infected immature mice, ILC2s culture for analysis through ELISA, qPCR, proliferation assay and immunofluorescence. We also describe a method for adoptive transfer of ILC2s in naïve immature mice to determine the causal relationship of ILC2s with aiway disease.

2 Materials

2.1 Animals and Virus

1. BALB/c mice (Jackson Laboratory, Bar Harbor, ME).
2. RVA1B (ATCC, Manassas, Virginia).

2.2 Reagents

1. DPBS without calcium and magnesium (cat. no. 14190144, Gibco, Billings, Montana).
2. DPBS with calcium and magnesium (cat. no. 14040117, Gibco, Billings, Montana).
3. DMEM (cat. no. 11965084, Gibco, Billings, Montana).
4. Penicillin-Streptomycin (cat. no. 15070063, Gibco, Billings, Montana).
5. UltraPure 0.5 M EDTA, pH 8.0 (cat. no. 15575020, Carlsbad, CA).
6. Collagenase IV (cat. No. LS004186, Worthington, Columbus, OH).
7. DNase I (cat. No. LS006342, Worthington, Columbus, OH).
8. RBC lysis buffer (cat. no. 00-4333-57, Invitrogen, Carlsbad, CA).
9. Trypan Blue Solution (cat. no. 1525006, Gibco, Billings, Montana).
10. Bovine Serum Albumin (cat. no. A3912, Sigma Aldrich, St. Louis, MO).
11. Pacific Blue™ Succinimidyl Ester (cat. no. P10163, Molecular Probes, Eugene, OR).
12. DMSO (cat. no. D2650, Sigma-Aldrich, St. Louis, MO).
13. 1 M Tris-HCI Buffer, pH 7.5 (cat. no. 15567027, Invitrogen, Carlsbad, CA)
14. Formaldehyde (cat. no. F79-1, Fisher Scientific, Waltham, MA).

15. Streptavidin Microbeads (cat. no.130-090-485, Miltenyi Biotech).
16. DAPI (4′,6-diamidino-2-phenylindole, cat. no. D21490, Invitrogen, Carlsbad, CA).
17. RPMI-1640 (cat. no. 1875093, Gibco, Billings, Montana).
18. IL-13 ELISA kit (Cat. no. 88–7137-22, Invitrogen, Carlsbad, CA).
19. RNAeasy Micro and Mini Kit (cat. no. 74004 and 74104, respectively, Qiagen, Gaithersburg, MD).
20. Bromodeoxyuridine (BrdU, cat. no. B5002, Sigma-Aldrich, St. Louis, MO).
21. Carboxyfluorescein diacetate succinimidyl ester (CFSE; cat. no. C1157, Molecular Probes, Eugene, OR).
22. IL-2, IL-7, IL-25 and IL-33 (R&D, Minneapolis, MN).
23. BrdU (cat. no. B5002-100MG, Sigma-Aldrich, St. Louis, MO).
24. ProLong Gold-Antifade Mountant with DAPI (Thermo Fisher Scientific, Waltham, MA).

2.3 Antibodies

Anti-mouse CD16/32 (cat. no. 101302), FITC anti-mouse lineage cocktail (CD3ε, Gr-1/Ly-6G/Ly-6C, CD11b, B220/CD45R, Ter-119, cat. no. 133302), FITC-conjugated anti-CD11C (cat. no. 117306), FITC anti-FcεRIα (cat. no. 134306), FITC anti-T-cell receptor-β (TCRβ) (cat. no. 109206), FITC anti-F4/80 (cat. no. 123108), peridinin-chlorophyll-protein complex (PerCP)-cyanin5.5 (Cy5.5) anti-CD25 (cat. no. 101912), allophycocyanin (APC) anti-CD127 (cat. no. 121122), biotin anti-mouse TER-119 (Cat. no., 116,204, Biolegend), biotin anti-mouse/human CD11b (Cat. no. 101204), biotin anti-mouse Ly-6G/Ly-6C (Gr-1) (Cat. no. 108404), biotin anti-Mouse CD3e (Cat. no. 100304), biotin anti-Mouse CD45R/B220 (Cat. no. 103204), biotin anti-Mouse TCRβ (Cat. no. 109204), biotin anti-Mouse FcεRIα (Cat. no. 134304), biotin anti-Mouse F4/80 (Cat. no. 123106) and biotin anti-Mouse CD11c (Cat. no. 117304) antibodies. All the above antibodies were purchased from BioLegend, San Diego, CA. Alexa Fluor 555-conjugated anti-BrdU antibody was purchased from Life Technologies, Waltham, MA.

2.4 Equipment

1. Dissecting scissors.
2. Forceps of various sizes, including 10 cm size.
3. 5 mL syringe (cat. no. 309646, BD Biosciences, San Jose, CA)
4. Tube rotator.
5. 1.5, 15 and 50-mL tubes

6. Cell strainer (cat. no. CLS431751, Corning, NY).
7. 5 mL polystyrene round-bottomed FACS tubes
8. Hemocytometer.
9. MS column (cat. no. 130-042-20, Miltenyi Biotech, Gaithersburg, MD).
10. MiniMACS separator (cat. no. 130-042-102, Miltenyi Biotech, Gaithersburg, MD).
11. Flow cytometer: LS Fortessa for flow cytometry and FACS Aria II (BD Biosciences, San Jose, CA) for cell sorting.
12. 96-well microplates, round bottom (cat. no. CLS3367, Corning, NY)
13. CO_2 incubator.

3 Methods

3.1 Lung Cell Preparation

1. Treat six-day-old BALB/c mice through the intranasal route under Forane anesthesia with RVA1B (20 μL of 1×10^8 plaque-forming units (pfu)/mL viral stock) or an equal volume of sham HeLa cell lysate.
2. One week post infection, sacrifice the mice and harvest the whole lung after perfusions with DPBS containing 5 mM EDTA. Transfer to 5 mL of ice-cold DMEM containing 1× Penicillin-Streptomycin (P/S). Keep on ice.
3. Digest the lungs in ice-cold DMEM containing 1× P/S, 10 mg/mL collagenase IV and 1 μg/mL DNase I for an hour on a rotator at room temperature (*see* **Note 1**).
4. Make a single-cell suspension by passing through a cell strainer while mincing the tissue on top of the strainer with flat end of 1 mL pipette tip.
5. Wash the strainer with ice-cold DMEM containing 10% FBS and 1× P/S, and combine the flow through.
6. Centrifuge cells at 200× *g* at 4 °C for 10 mins.
7. Resuspend in 1 mL of serum free DMEM containing 1× P/S.

3.2 Spleen Cell Preparation

1. Harvest the spleen and make single-cell suspension by mincing and passing through a cell strainer (*see* **Note 2**).
2. Wash the strainer with 5 mL of ice-cold DMEM containing 10% FBS and 1× P/S, and combine the flow-through.
3. Centrifuge the cells at 200× *g* at 4 °C for 10 mins.
4. Resuspend in 1 mL of ice-cold DMEM containing 1× P/S.

3.3 RBC Lysis

1. Add 1 mL of 1× RBC lysis buffer and resuspend the pellet. Incubate for 10 mins at room temperature.
2. Add 9 mL of DPBS to the tube at the end of the RBC lysis reaction.
3. Centrifuge the tubes at 200× *g* at 4 °C for 10 mins.
4. Resuspend cells in 1 mL of serum-free DMEM containing 1× P/S.
5. Pass the cell suspension through a 70 μm cell strainer.
6. Count the live cells using 0.4% Trypan blue solution.
7. Determine the total cell number of lung cell suspension. Keep aside the spleen cells on ice (*see* **Note 3**).
8. Transfer 2 mL total of lung cells (e.g., if having 10 lung samples, then add 200 μL from each sample) to the spleen cell suspension; spin all the cell suspensions at 200×*g* at 4 °C for 5 mins.
9. Resuspend each lung cell preparation in 100 μL of blocking buffer (DMEM, 1% FBS, 1% BSA and 1× P/S) and transfer to 1.5 mL tubes. Resuspend spleen cells mixed with lung cells into 1 mL of blocking buffer. Transfer 100 μL each into 1.5 mL tubes labelled 1 through 8.

3.4 Flow Cytometry Staining and Analysis of Lung ILC2s

1. Keep the tube no. 1 and 2 on ice. Set the heating block at 55 ° C. Add 1 μL of anti-mouse CD16/32 antibody to the rest of the tubes to block nonspecific binding to Fc receptors, followed by an FITC-conjugated antibody cocktail for lineage markers (CD3ε, Gr-1/Ly-6G/Ly-6C, CD11b, B220/CD45R, Ter-119), FITC anti-CD11C, FITC anti-FcεRIα, FITC anti-T-cell receptor-β (TCRβ) and FITC anti-F4/80 antibodies. To identify ILC2s, add PerCP-Cy5.5 anti-CD25 and APC anti-CD127 antibodies. Incubate on ice in the dark for 20 mins. In the meantime, put the tube no. 2 at 55 °C in heating block for 15 mins.
2. Remove tube no. 2 from heating block after 15 mins.
3. Add 1 mL cold DPBS (without calcium and magnesium) to all the tubes except tube no. 1 and centrifuge at 200× *g* at 4 °C for 5 mins.
4. Resuspend the pellet in 500 μL of DPBS (without calcium and magnesium). Add pacific blue dye (1 μg/mL in DMSO) to all the tubes except for tube no. 1, mix and incubate on ice for 10 mins in dark.
5. Spin the tubes at 200× *g* at 4 °C for 5 mins.
6. Aspirate the supernatant and resuspend the pellet in 200 μL of DPBS (without calcium and magnesium) containing 10 mM Tris, pH 7.4 to quench the reaction. Add another

800 μL of DPBS containing 10 mM Tris, pH 7.4, mix and incubate on ice in dark for 10–20 mins.

7. Spin the tubes at 200× *g* at 4 °C for 5 mins.
8. Resuspend the pellet in 400 μL 2% paraformaldehyde. Incubate at room temperature for 15 mins. Wash the cells once with DPBS and keep on ice.
9. Proceed with flow cytometry analysis by first selecting cells within the lymphocyte gate on the basis of forward-scatter (FSC) and side-scatter (SSC) properties. Gate out dead cells on the basis of pacific blue staining. ILC2s can be identified as Lineage– CD25+ CD127+ [9].

3.5 Preparation of ILC2s Staining from Multiple Mice for Sorting

3.5.1 Staining with Biotin Labelled Antibodies for Depletion of Lineage Positive Cells

1. Follow the lung sample preparation as described above but pool the lungs from 6 to 10 mice into a single tube and proceed with collagenase IV digestion and RBC lysis.
2. Following RBC lysis, resuspend lung cells and spleen cells in 1 mL of blocking buffer.
3. Transfer 100 μL of lung cells to spleen cell suspension and spin all the cell suspensions at 200× *g* at 4 °C for 5 mins (*see* **Note 4**).
4. Resuspend the cells in 1 mL of blocking buffer containing anti-mouse CD16/CD32 antibody to block nonspecific binding to Fc receptors. Label cells with the biotin-conjugated anti-mouse antibodies for staining of lineage-positive cells. Add antibodies as follows:

Biotin anti-MouseTer-119	[2 μL (10^6 cells), 4 μL(10^7), 40 μL(10^8)]
Biotin anti-mouse CD11b	[2 μL (10^6 cells), 4 μL(10^7), 40 μL(10^8)]
Biotin anti-Mouse Ly6G/Ly6C (Gr-1)	[2 μL (10^6 cells), 4 μL(10^7), 40 μL(10^8)]
Biotin anti-Mouse CD3e	[2 μL (10^6 cells), 4 μL(10^7), 40 μL(10^8)]
Biotin anti-Mouse CD45R/B220	[2 μL (10^6 cells), 4 μL(10^7), 40 μL(10^8)]
Biotin anti-Mouse TCRβ	[1 μL (10^6), 10 μL(10^7), or 10 μL(10^8]
Biotin anti-Mouse FcεRIα	[1 μL (10^6), 1 μL(10^7) or 1 μL(10^8)]
Biotin anti-Mouse F4/80	[1 μL (10^6), 2.5 μL (10^7) or 25 μL(10^8]
Biotin anti-Mouse CD11c	[1 μL (10^6), 2.5 μL(10^7) or 25 μL(10^8)]

5. Stain cells by keeping on ice for 15 mins.

6. Wash cells by adding 10 mL of DPBS without calcium and magnesium containing 1% BSA (buffer 1) per 10^8 cells and centrifuge at 200× *g* at 4 °C for 5 mins. Aspirate supernatant completely.
7. Resuspend cells in 700 μL of buffer 1 per 10^8 cells.
8. Add 200 μL of streptavidin microbeads per 10^8 cells.
9. Mix well and refrigerate the cells for 15 mins (4–8 °C). Do not place them on ice.
10. Wash cells by adding 10 mL of Buffer 1 per 10^8 cells and centrifuge at 200× *g* at 4 °C for 10 mins. Aspirate supernatant completely.
11. Resuspend cells in 1 mL of DPBS without calcium and magnesium containing 0.5% BSA and 2 mM EDTA (Buffer 2).

3.5.2 Magnetic Separation

1. Place the MS column in the magnetic field of MiniMACS separator.
2. Prepare column by rinsing with 500 μL of buffer 2.
3. Apply cell suspension onto the column. Collect flow-through containing unlabeled cells.
4. Wash column with 3 times with 500 μL of buffer 2. Collect unlabeled cells that pass through and combine with the effluent.
5. Spin down the unlabeled cells.
6. Resuspend cells in 1 mL of blocking buffer.
7. Count cells numbers.

3.5.3 Fluorescence-Activated Cell Sorting of Lung ILC2s

1. Proceed with cell surface staining of ILC2s using the antibodies against lineage markers, CD25 and CD127. Instead of Pacific blue, at the end of staining, add DAPI at a final concentration of 0.1 μg/mL to 500 μL of cell suspension in DPBS with calcium and magnesium.
2. Carry out flow cytometry analysis as described above.
3. To sort ILC2s, set the sorting gate to include live lymphoid cells in the Lineage– CD25+ CD127+ gate.
4. To sort lineage positive cells as negative controls, set the sorting gate to include live lymphoid cells in the Lineage+ gate.
5. Collect the sorted cells in 15 mL tubes pre-coated with 5% BSA (*see* **Note 5**)

3.6 In Vitro Culture of ILC2s

1. Centrifuge the sorted ILC2s at 200× *g* at 4°C for 10 mins and resuspend in RPMI containing 10% FBS, 1× P/S, 10 mM HEPES, 1× NEAA and a combination of IL-2, IL-7, IL-25,

and IL-33 (10 ng/mL) as per the experiment requirements (*see* **Note 6**) [9].

2. Plate the ILC2s at 5–6 × 10^3 cells/100 μL in round-bottom 96-well plates.
3. After 1–3 days of stimulation, centrifuge the plates at 200× *g* and test the supernatants for IL-13 with ELISA.
4. Extract the RNA from the cell pellet using RNeasy Micro Kit (*see* **Note 7**).
5. Synthesize the cDNA and subject to quantitative PCR (qPCR) for IL-13, IL-5, ST2L, IL-17, IL-17RB, and GATA3 [9].

3.7 Cell Proliferation and Immunofluorescence Analysis of ILC2

1. Dissolve 100 mg of bromodeoxyuridine (BrdU) in 32.5 mL of anhydrous DMSO. Dilute 10 μL of this 10 mM stock solution in 10 mL of 37 °C tissue culture medium to make a 10 μM labeling solution.
2. Centrifuge the 96 wells plates containing cells at 200 × *g* for 5 mins. Remove culture medium from cells and replace with BrdU labeling solution (*see* **Note 8**).
3. Incubate cells at 37 °C for 24 h.
4. Centrifuge the 96 wells plates containing cells at 200 × *g* for 5 mins.
5. Remove labeling solution and wash once with 300 μL HBSS containing 5mM HEPES.
6. Centrifuge at 200 × *g* for 5 mins, remove HBSS and add 1 mL of 3.7% formaldehyde in HBSS containing 5mM HEPES to each well.
7. Incubate for 15 mins at room temperature.
8. Wash with HBSS containing 5mM HEPES 2 ×, 2 mins each and transfer the cells on slides via cytospin.
9. Mark around the cells with hydrophobic barrier pen and add 1 mL of Triton® ×-100 permeabilization buffer (0.3% Triton ×-100 in HBSS containing 5mM HEPES).
10. Incubate for 20 mins at room temperature.
11. Remove the permeabilization buffer and add 200 μl of 1 N HCl.
12. Incubate for 10 mins on ice.
13. Remove the solution and add 1 mL of 2 N HCl.
14. Incubate for 10 mins at room temperature.
15. Add 200 μ phosphate/citric acid buffer, pH 7.4 (182 mL of 0.2 M Na_2HPO_4 and 18 mL 0.1 M citric acid).

16. Incubate for 10 mins at room temperature.
17. Wash with Triton® ×-100 permeabilization buffer, 3x, 2 mins each.
18. Remove the solution and add alexa fluor 555-conjugated anti-BrdU antibody in DPBS containing 1% BSA.
19. Incubate overnight at room temperature.
20. Wash with Triton® ×-100 permeabilization buffer, 3 x, 5 mins each.
21. Mount the slides using ProLong Gold-Antifade Mountant with DAPI.
22. Image cells with appropriate filters using a fluorescence microscope.

3.8 Adoptive Transfer of ILC2s

1. Centrifuge the sorted ILC2s at 200× *g* at 4°C for 10 mins and resuspend in RPMI containing 10% FBS, 1× P/S, 10 mM HEPES, 1× NEAA and 10 μM carboxyfluorescein diacetate succinimydyl methyl ester (CFSE). Incubate for 15 mins at 37 °C in a cell culture incubator.
2. Centrifuge at 200× *g*; resuspend to 1–3 × 10^4 cells/20 μL in DPBS with calcium and magnesium. Keep on ice. Intranasally transfer 20 μL volume into each pup under forane anesthesia (*see* **Note 9**). As negative controls, transfer the sorted lineage positive cells in a similar manner.
3. Harvest the lungs 24 h later by perfusing through the pulmonary artery with DPBS containing 5 mM EDTA, fixing with 10% phosphate buffered formalin overnight and paraffin embedding.
4. Section the parafin blocks at 500 μm intervals at a thickness of 5 μM.
5. Deparaffinize the section, hydrate and mount with using Pro-Long Gold-Antifade Mountant with DAPI.
6. Visualize the CFSE labelled ILC2s in the lungs using fluorescence microscope.
7. If the adoptive transfer is successful, harvest the rest of the lungs 14 days post adoptive transfer, since we previously observed mucus metaplasia 2 weeks after maximal ILC2 expansion [10].
8. Process the lungs for qPCR, histology and immunofluorescence analysis.

4 Notes

1. The time of lung digestion is critical for the recovery of cells from the preparation. The digestion process should not exceed the recommended time or may require optimization to avoid cell death and clumping.
2. The spleen does not require digestion with collagenase. The cells can be recovered directly by mincing the spleens on the cell strainer while adding ice cold DMEM complete medium. Using collagenase will lead to cell death and clumping.
3. 10^6–10^7 cells are recommended for flow cytometry. Since the ILC2s are rare, using lesser lung cells will not show clear population.
4. It is important to have initial cell numbers of 10^7–10^8 for sorting, otherwise, not enough ILC2s will be obtained.
5. Pre-coating tubes with 5% BSA helps to reduce the static charge and deflection of cells towards the walls of the tubes.
6. IL-2 and IL-7 are used for maintenance of ILC2s in culture, however activation and rapid proliferation may require the use of IL-25 and IL-33.
7. It is recommended that RNA isolation kit designed for purifying RNA from small number of cells ($<10^5$) be used in order to achieve maximum recovery of RNA.
8. The media should be removed from the well using a 200μl pipette and should not be aspirated.
9. We observed that 3×10^4 ILC2s are sufficient to induce mucus metaplasia in neonatal mice. Using lesser ILC2s may not result in desired phenotype.

References

1. Kotaniemi-Syrjanen A et al (2003) Rhinovirus-induced wheezing in infancy – the first sign of childhood asthma? J Allergy Clin Immunol 111(1):66–71
2. Lemanske RF Jr et al (2005) Rhinovirus illnesses during infancy predict subsequent childhood wheezing. J Allergy Clin Immunol 116(3):571–577
3. Jackson DJ et al (2008) Wheezing rhinovirus illnesses in early life predict asthma development in high-risk children. Am J Respir Crit Care Med 178(7):667–672
4. Carroll KN et al (2009) Season of infant bronchiolitis and estimates of subsequent risk and burden of early childhood asthma. J Allergy Clin Immunol 123(4):964–966
5. Han M et al (2017) The innate cytokines IL-25, IL-33, and TSLP cooperate in the induction of type 2 innate lymphoid cell expansion and mucous metaplasia in rhinovirus-infected immature mice. J Immunol 199(4): 1308–1318
6. Halim TY et al (2012) Lung natural helper cells are a critical source of Th2 cell-type cytokines in protease allergen-induced airway inflammation. Immunity 36(3):451–463
7. Klein Wolterink RG et al (2013) Essential, dose-dependent role for the transcription factor Gata3 in the development of IL-5+ and IL-13+ type 2 innate lymphoid cells. Proc Natl Acad Sci USA 110(25):10240–10245

8. Wong SH et al (2012) Transcription factor RORalpha is critical for nuocyte development. Nat Immunol 13(3):229–236
9. Rajput C, Cui T, Han M, Lei J, Hinde JL, Wu Q, Bentley JK, Hershenson MB (2017) RORalpha-dependent type 2 innate lymphoid cells are required and sufficient for mucous metaplasia in immature mice. Am J Physiol Lung Cell Mol Physiol 312(6):L983–L993
10. Hong JY et al (2014) Neonatal rhinovirus induces mucous metaplasia and airways hyper-responsiveness through IL-25 and type 2 innate lymphoid cells. J Allergy Clin Immunol 134(2):429–439

Chapter 13

Assessment of Rhinovirus Infection in a Mouse Model of COPD

Krist H. Antunes, Millie M. Jackson, Kyle T. Mincham, Robert J. Snelgrove, and Aran Singanayagam

Abstract

A better understanding of the mechanisms governing virus-induced exacerbations of chronic obstructive pulmonary disease (COPD) is urgently needed to develop more effective therapeutic approaches. Animal models are invaluable tools for gaining mechanistic insight into innate immunity. Here, we describe the methods required to establish a short-term mouse model comprising elastase administration to induce features of COPD, combined with infection using the minor group rhinovirus serotype A1 (RV-A1). This model recapitulates the hallmark features of human virus-induced COPD exacerbation and facilitates the study of mechanisms that drive these episodes.

Key words Chronic obstructive pulmonary disease, Innate immunity, Elastase, Emphysema, Bronchoalveolar lavage, Inflammation

1 Introduction

Chronic obstructive pulmonary disease (COPD) is an inflammatory condition characterized by irreversible airflow limitation that is one of the leading causes of death worldwide [1]. The disease is punctuated by periods of symptomatic worsening (termed "exacerbations") which are associated with accelerated disease progression and mortality. Around 47–56% of COPD exacerbations are triggered by respiratory viruses, most commonly rhinoviruses (RV) [2]. Due to the significant clinical, social, and financial burden of COPD exacerbations, understanding the mechanisms driving these episodes is of paramount importance to facilitate the development of more effective prevention and treatment strategies.

Experimental human challenge studies in individuals with COPD have confirmed a causal role for RVs in precipitating exacerbations [3]. However, the mechanisms underlying RV-induced COPD exacerbations remain poorly understood. One key approach

Umadevi Sajjan (ed.), *Rhinovirus: Methods and Protocols*, Methods in Molecular Biology, vol. 2903,
https://doi.org/10.1007/978-1-0716-4410-2_13,

to understanding these mechanisms is to employ animal models of exacerbated COPD which then allow the use of experimental manipulations to block or augment immune pathways and gain understanding of causally important disease mechanisms. Models of COPD in small animals such as mice, rats, and guinea pigs are varied and include exposure to cigarette smoke, inflammatory stimuli (e.g., lipopolysaccharide), proteolytic enzymes (e.g., elastase), or genetic modification [4]. In some instances, these inducers can be used in combination [5]. Some of these models (such as cigarette smoke) require repeated exposures over a long period and are therefore time-consuming, impractical, and expensive. We have developed a short-term mouse model combining intranasal administration of a single dose of porcine pancreatic elastase followed by infection with the minor group virus RV-A1 10 days later. This model recapitulates the hallmark features of human COPD exacerbation, including baseline histological emphysema and exacerbated inflammation/mucus secretion following viral infection [6]. The model therefore facilitates the study of viral-induced exacerbations and allows identification of mechanisms driving dysregulated host immune responses occurring during these episodes, as demonstrated in a number of recent publications [7–10].

2 Materials

2.1 Reagents Required for Elastase Preparation

1. Elastase, Porcine Pancreas, High Purity, Crystallized (Merck Millipore catalog number 324682-250 U).
2. Sterile water for reconstitution.
3. Sterile phosphate buffer saline (without calcium and magnesium) for dilution to the required concentration.

2.2 Cells and Reagents Required for RV Growth and Purification

1. RV serotype A1 (RV-A1) (American Type Tissue Culture Collection (ATCC VR-1366).
2. H1 HeLa Cells (ATCC CRL-1958).
3. Dulbecco's modified eagle medium (DMEM) supplemented with 10% (for initial cell culture) or 2% (infection medium) fetal calf serum (FCS), 2% HEPES buffer 1 M, and 1% sodium bicarbonate.
4. 175 cm^2 culture flasks
5. 0.2 μm syringe filter
6. Polyethylene glycol (PEG) 6000.
7. 5 M sodium chloride solution
8. Amicon ultracentrifugal device 100,000 NMCO (Merck Millipore).

2.3 Reagents Required for Intranasal Dosing of Mice and Downstream Pulmonary Immune Analysis

1. Isofluorane (anesthesia for intranasal administration).
2. Pentobarbitone solution (anesthesia for euthanasia).
3. Sterile PBS for bronchoalveolar lavage.
4. Roswell Park Memorial Institute (RPMI) medium supplemented with 10% FCS.
5. 4% paraformaldehyde (lung fixation for histology)
6. RNeasy kit for RNA extraction (Qiagen).
7. Omniscript RT kit for reverse transcription of RNA to cDNA (Qiagen).

3 Methods

3.1 Preparation of Porcine Pancreatic Elastase

Reconstitute lyophilized elastase at a concentration of 10 mg/mL in sterile water and store aliquots at −80 °C. Enzymatic activity varies according to batch and is recorded on an accompanying datasheet (*see* **Note 1**). When required for an experiment, dilute stock solution in PBS to a final concentration of 24 units/mL (1.2 units in 50 uL). Mix by manual inversion (*see* **Note 2**). Keep on ice until intranasal dose administration in mice.

3.2 Cell Culture for Rhinovirus Growth

1. Cell culture and RV infection: Culture H1HeLa cells (~ passage 2–7) in 175 cm^2 culture flasks using DMEM medium supplemented with 10% FCS and maintain at 37 °C with 5% CO_2. When cells are ~90% confluent, wash the cells twice with 10 mL of DMEM with 2% FCS medium and infect with RV-A1 in 20 mL of 2% DMEM medium. Shake flasks gently on an orbital shaker at room temperature for 1 h and then incubate at 37 °C with 5% CO_2 until 100% cytopathic effect (CPE) is observed by light microscopy (~18–24 h).
2. RV growth and harvesting: Dislodge the infected cells manually (thrust hand against the outer aspect of the flask). Transfer all cells into a single 175 cm^2 flask. Lyse cells to release virus particles by performing freeze/thawing twice (in a −80 °C freezer or on dry ice). Transfer the infected cell-media suspension to a 50 mL centrifuge tube and centrifuge at 2500× *g* for 15 mins at 4 °C to pellet cell debris. Remove the supernatant and add it to 500 mL of 2% DMEM medium. Filter through a 0.2 μm syringe filter.
3. Add 15–20 mL of filtered virus per flask to H1Hela cells cultured to 90% confluence in 25 × 175 cm^2 flasks (25 flasks are required to ensure a sufficient quantity of virus is generated). Shake flasks gently using an orbital shaker at room temperature for 1 h, then add a further 5 mL of 2% DMEM

medium before incubating at 37 °C with 5% CO_2 until 100% CPE observed by light microscopy (~18–24 h).

4. Dislodge cells manually (thrust hand against the outer aspect of the flask) and use a sterile cell scraper to remove any adherent cells. Collect all cells in 12 × 50 mL centrifuge tubes. Centrifuge at 380 x g for 15 mins to pellet.
5. Discard the supernatant and resuspend the pellet in 5 mL of sterile PBS and combine into a single 50 mL centrifuge tube. Centrifuge at 2700× *g* for 15 mins to pellet. Repeat the wash step using 50 mL of sterile PBS, followed by centrifugation to pellet cells. Resuspend in a final volume of 36 mL of PBS.

3.3 Rhinovirus Purification

1. Freeze-thaw the 36 mL solution twice, then centrifuge at 2700× *g* to pellet debris. Filter the supernatant through a 0.2 μm syringe filter.
2. Precipitate the virus from the supernatant by dissolving 2.8 g Polyethylene Glycol-6000 and 4 mL of 5 M NaCl into the solution, followed by incubation on ice for 1 h with gentle inversion every 15 mins.
3. Centrifuge at 2500× g for 1 h to pellet the virus. Remove the supernatant and dissolve the pellet in 15 mL of PBS on a roller, followed by centrifugation at 4000 rpm for 15 min to remove debris.
4. Purify and concentrate the virus using a 0.2 μm syringe filter in a 100,000 MWCO 15 mL Amicon ultracentrifugal device, centrifuging at 2000× *g* until the volume is reduced to around 500 μL. Discard the flow-through. Add a further 10 mL of PBS and mix with pipette before repeating centrifugation. Concentrate virus preparation by centrifugation at 2000× *g* down to 500 uL again. Remove the concentrated virus and add a further 2 mL of PBS to the ultracentrifugal device to wash out any remaining virus particles. Combine this with the 500 μL concentrated virus to give a total preparation volume of 2.5–3 mL and store at −80 °C (*see* **Note 3**).

3.4 Intranasal Administration of Elastase and Rhinovirus Infection of Mice

1. Purchase 8–10-week-old female C57BL/6 mice and house within individually ventilated cages in specific pathogen-free conditions.
2. For intranasal administration of elastase (or PBS as control), lightly anesthetize mouse with inhaled isoflurane and oxygen at 2 litres/minute administered via an induction chamber.
3. Closely monitor mice. Once respiratory rate starts to slow, remove mouse from chamber (*see* **Note 4**) and administer 1.2 units of porcine pancreatic elastase in 50 μL PBS intranasally using a pipette.

4. Leave mice for 10 days to allow COPD-like changes to develop.
5. After 10 days, intranasally infect mice (using a similar technique to Subheading 3.4, **step 3**) with 50 μL of purified virus (2×10^6 $TCID_{50}$/mL) or ultraviolet (UV)-inactivated RV control (by irradiation with 1200 μJ/cm^2 UV light for 30 min using a UV crosslinker).
6. Euthanize mice at time points of interest post-infection by intraperitoneal injection of 0.2 mL of 20% pentobarbitone solution.

3.5 Assessment of Lung Histology and Immune Responses

1. *Bronchoalveolar lavage (BAL):* After euthanasia, expose the trachea by dissection. Use a needle to insert a small hole into superior aspect of the trachea and insert a plastic cannula. Insert and aspirate back 1.5 mL of PBS four times and store in a microcentrifuge tube. Centrifuge the recovered BAL fluid at 2000× *g* for 5 min at room temperature. Remove the supernatant and store it at −80 °C for the quantification of immune mediators and cytokine proteins. Resuspend the cell pellet in 500 μL of 10% RPMI medium and analyze cellular inflammation, including eosinophils, neutrophils, and macrophages, using flow cytometry or cytospin.
2. *Lung histology:* Following animal sacrifice, dissect the thoracic cavity to expose the heart and lungs. Perfuse the lungs via injection of PBS through the heart using a 21-gauge needle and inflate with 4% paraformaldehyde (PFA). Remove the lungs and fix them in 4% PFA for 24 h at 4 °C. Transfer the lung to microtubes containing 70% ethanol. Embed in 4% paraffin. Cut 5 μm thick sagittal sections using a microtome. Leave at 4 °C until processing. Sections can be mounted on slides and stained with hematoxylin and eosin to visualize lung morphology and cellular inflammatory infiltrates and periodic acid Schiff to visualize mucus. Alveolar chord length can be determined by measuring the diameter of air spaces in 10 random fields per slide (*see* **Note 5**). Representative images from untreated mice and mice treated with elastase are presented in Fig. 1. The elastase-treated mice show extensive emphysema.
3. *Lung tissue for qPCR:* Remove the right apical lobe and store it in 200 μL RNA protection buffer for 24 h at 4 °C, followed by longer-term storage at −80 °C. Extract RNA by homogenizing lung lobe followed by extraction using the RNeasy kit (Qiagen) according to the manufacturers' instructions. Convert to cDNA using the Omniscript RT kit (Qiagen) for downstream qPCR assays to quantify the expression of immune genes of interest.

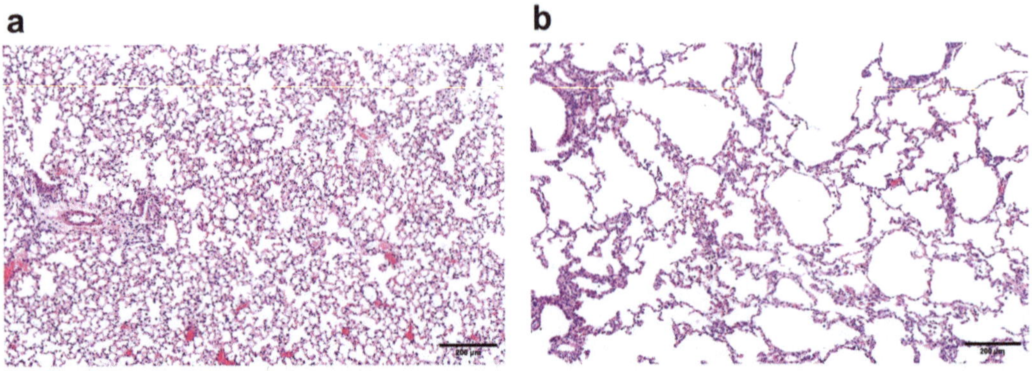

Fig. 1 Histological evaluation in elastase model of COPD. C57BL/6 mice were challenged with a single dose of procine pancreatic elatase or PBS as control. At 10 days post-challenge, lungs were formalin-fixed, paraffin-embedded and stained with haematoxylin and eosin. Representative images of mice treated with (**a**) PBS and (**b**) elastase

4 Notes

1. Accompanying datasheet has information about both activity and specific activity of the elastase batch. Activity rather than specific activity should be used for calculating dose. Use of specific activity will lead to underdosing.
2. Mix by gentle manual inversion. Avoid vigorously vortexing or shaking the elastase solution, as this may diminish enzymatic activity.
3. Avoid prolonged periods of storage of purified RV at −80 °C as degradation and reduction in infectious titer may occur. Ideally, batches should be used within months of preparation.
4. C57BL/6 mice can be difficult to administer an intranasal dose due to a narrower window between under- and over-anesthetization compared to other mouse strains. Use of a stopwatch timer can circumvent this problem by ensuring that a consistent amount of time in the induction chamber is maintained.
5. As only a single dose of 50 μL of elastase is administered, histological changes may not be uniformly distributed throughout all lobes equally. If the requirement is to model more widespread changes to mimic severe emphysema, repeated dose administrations may be required.

Acknowledgments

The authors acknowledge financial support from Imperial College London through an Imperial College Research Fellowship grant awarded to K.T.M. Parts of this work were also funded through a Rosetrees Trust/The Stoneygate Trust Project Grant (PGS21/10072). R.J.S. is a Wellcome Trust Senior Fellow in Basic Biomedical Sciences (209458/Z/17/Z). A.S. is a Medical Research Council Clinician Scientist Fellow (MR/V000098/1).

References

1. Christenson SA, Smith BM, Bafadhel M, Putcha N (2022) Chronic obstructive pulmonary disease. Lancet 399(10342):2227–2242
2. Singanayagam A, Joshi PV, Mallia P, Johnston SL (2012) Viruses exacerbating chronic pulmonary disease: the role of immune modulation. BMC Med 10:27
3. Mallia P, Message SD, Gielen V, Contoli M, Gray K, Kebadze T et al (2011) Experimental rhinovirus infection as a human model of chronic obstructive pulmonary disease exacerbation. Am J Respir Crit Care Med 183(6): 734–742
4. Ghorani V, Boskabady MH, Khazdair MR, Kianmeher M (2017) Experimental animal models for COPD: a methodological review. Tob Induc Dis 15:25
5. Sajjan U, Ganesan S, Comstock AT, Shim J, Wang Q, Nagarkar DR et al (2009) Elastase- and LPS-exposed mice display altered responses to rhinovirus infection. Am J Physiol Lung Cell Mol Physiol 297(5):L931–L944
6. Singanayagam A, Glanville N, Walton RP, Aniscenko J, Pearson RM, Pinkerton JW et al (2015) A short-term mouse model that reproduces the immunopathological features of rhinovirus-induced exacerbation of COPD. Clin Sci (Lond) 129(3):245–258
7. Singanayagam A, Glanville N, Girkin JL, Ching YM, Marcellini A, Porter JD et al (2018) Corticosteroid suppression of antiviral immunity increases bacterial loads and mucus production in COPD exacerbations. Nat Commun 9(1): 2229
8. Singanayagam A, Glanville N, Cuthbertson L, Bartlett NW, Finney LJ, Turek E et al (2019) Inhaled corticosteroid suppression of cathelicidin drives dysbiosis and bacterial infection in chronic obstructive pulmonary disease. Sci Transl Med 11(507)
9. Finney LJ, Glanville N, Farne H, Aniscenko J, Fenwick P, Kemp SV et al (2020) Inhaled corticosteroids downregulate the SARS-CoV-2 receptor ACE2 in COPD through suppression of type I interferon. J Allergy Clin Immunol
10. Singanayagam A, Footitt J, Marczynski M, Radicioni G, Cross MT, Finney LJ et al (2022) Airway mucins promote immunopathology in virus-exacerbated chronic obstructive pulmonary disease. J Clin Invest

Chapter 14

Infection of Immature Mice with Rhinovirus for the Study of Asthma Pathogenesis

Mingyuan Han and Marc Hershenson

Abstract

Early-life wheezing-associated respiratory infection with rhinovirus (RV) is a risk factor for asthma development in combination with allergen sensitization and family history. RV infection of immature mice is a useful model to decipher potential immunological mechanisms underlying asthma development following RV infection. Increased type 2 immune response, expansion of group 2 innate lymphoid cells (ILC2s), eosinophilic inflammation, mucous metaplasia, and airway hyperresponsiveness have been observed in RV-infected six-day-old mice. Herein, we present several materials and methods used for propagating and partially purifying RV, measuring RV titers, infecting immature mice with RV, and harvesting lung tissue for whole lung mRNA extraction and flow cytometry.

Key words Asthma, Early-life, Mouse, Methods, Rhinovirus, Type 2 immune response, Group 2 innate lymphoid cells (ILC2s)

1 Introduction

Rhinoviruses (RVs) are small positive-strand RNA viruses grouped into the family Picornaviridae [1]. First identified in the 1950s, RV infections are recognized as the most common cause of upper and lower respiratory tract infections [2, 3], as well as asthma- and chronic obstructive pulmonary disease (COPD)-associated exacerbations [4–6]. In addition, epidemiologic studies in high-risk infants with a family history of allergy indicate that early-life wheezing-associated respiratory tract infections by RVs are major risk factors for asthma development in combination with other factors such as allergen sensitization, microbiome, genetic factors, or environmental exposure [7–12]. However, it is unclear whether early-life rhinovirus infection causes asthma or whether RV preferably infects children who are predisposed to asthma development.

A minor group strain, RV-A1B, which attaches to proteins of the low-density lipoprotein receptor (LDL-R) as an entry receptor

Umadevi Sajjan (ed.), *Rhinovirus: Methods and Protocols*, Methods in Molecular Biology, vol. 2903,
https://doi.org/10.1007/978-1-0716-4410-2_14,

[13, 14], has been employed to infect adult mice intranasally as described elsewhere [15, 16]. Similarly, we have extended RV-A1B to infect six-day-old mice to establish the early-life infection model [17]. A prolonged type 2 immune response, featuring increased levels of IL-4, IL-5, and IL-13, as well as mucous metaplasia and airway hyperresponsiveness, occurs in RV-infected six-day-old immature mice but not in adult mice [17, 18]. The RV-induced asthma-like phenotype in immature mice is IL-13-dependent, and group 2 innate lymphoid cells (ILC2s), rather than TCR-β-positive cells, are the major cellular source of IL-13 [17, 18]. Further studies show that RV infection of six-day-old mice induces expression of epithelial-derived innate cytokines, IL-25, IL-33, and TSLP, each of which is all required for the maximal ILC2 expansion and functions, as well as the asthma-like phenotype [19].

The availability of an early-life RV infection murine model enables researchers to determine the role of cytokines (TSLP, IL-1β) [19, 20], innate immune signaling (inflammasome) [20, 21], and immune cells (ILC2s and macrophages) [22] by employing gene-specific and/or tissue-specific knockout mice, as well as developmental and strain differences in asthma development after viral infection [18, 21, 23]. Most recently, we found that early-life RV infection with RV-A1B alters the response to subsequent heterologous infection with RV-A2, including exaggerated type 2 inflammation, mucous metaplasia, and airway hyperresponsiveness [24]. This chapter will focuses on the methodology commonly used to propagate RV-A1B, infect mice with RV, and analyze mice after infection. All materials needed for these methods, along with suggested preparation and storage of these materials, are listed herein.

2 Materials

It is critical to perform all preparations in a biosafety cabinet to keep all materials used for H1HeLa cell culturing, plaque assay, and RV propagation sterile. This will help avoid contamination of culture media and H1HeLa cells to have the reliable quality of virus stock and accurate results for virus titration based on the methods listed below.

2.1 H1HeLa Cell Subculturing

1. Sterile tissue-culture-treated round culture dishes, 100 mm and 150 mm sizes.
2. H1HeLa cell (ATCC CRL-1958).
3. H1HeLa media: Dulbecco's minimal essential media (DMEM), 100 units/ml of penicillin, 100 μg/ml of streptomycin, 10% fetal bovine serum (FBS).
4. Phosphate-buffered saline (PBS), without calcium and magnesium.

5. Trypsin–EDTA: 0.25% trypsin, 0.9 mM EDTA, 0.025 mM phenol red in PBS.
6. Sterile polystyrene pipettes, 1-, 5-,10-, and 25-mL.
7. Waste container.
8. Cell culture incubator set at 37 °C, 5% CO_2.
9. Hemocytometer.
10. Trypan blue solution: 0.4% trypan blue dye in sterile PBS.

2.2 RV-A1B Propagation

1. H1HeLa cells with 90% confluence in 150 mm sterile tissue-culture-treated round culture dishes.
2. Phosphate-buffered saline (PBS), without calcium and magnesium.
3. RV-A1B propagation media: DMEM, 100 units/mL of penicillin, 100 μg/mL of streptomycin, 2 mM $MgCl_2$.
4. Rhinovirus A1B (ATCC VR-1645) master stock.
5. BSL-2 biosafety cabinet.
6. Cell culture incubator set at 33 °C, 5% CO_2.
7. Cell scraper.
8. −70 °C ultra-low freezers
9. Sterile 50-mL polypropylene conical tubes.

2.3 RV-A1B Concentration and Ultra-Filtration

1. Sterile 50-mL polypropylene conical tubes.
2. 10 μg/mL RNase A stock
3. 30,000 U/mL DNase 1 stock
4. Sterile 250 mL vacuum low protein-binding filter unit with 0.45 μm cellulose acetate membrane.
5. Millipore Amicon Stirred Cell (400 mL).
6. Millipore Ultracel 100 kDa NMW ultrafiltration discs (*see* **Note 1**).
7. 70% ethanol
8. Ice-cold, cell culture-grade, endotoxin-free PBS with Ca^{2+} and Mg^{2+}.
9. Nitrogen gas tank supplied with a pressure regulator and tubing system to connect the ultrafiltration unit to the nitrogen tank.
10. A magnetic stirring plate.
11. A refrigerated cold room (4 °C).
12. Cryogenic vials (2.0 mL).
13. −70 °C ultra-low freezers.

2.4 Plaque Assays for Viral Titer

1. Sterile tissue culture-treated polystyrene 6-well cell culture plate.
2. Sterile 50-mL polypropylene conical tubes.
3. H1HeLa cell (ATCC CRL-1958).
4. H1HeLa media: DMEM, 100 units/ml of penicillin, 100 μg/mL of streptomycin, 10% FBS.
5. Virus dilution media: DMEM, 100 units/ml of penicillin, 100 μg/mL of streptomycin.
6. Microcentrifuge tubes (1.5 mL).
7. Endotoxin-free PBS with calcium and magnesium.
8. 2% low melting point SeaPlaque GTG agarose: Dissolve 2 g of low melting point SeaPlaque GTG agarose in 100 mL of endotoxin-free PBS with Ca^{2+} and Mg^{2+} in a 500 mL glass ISO bottle. Autoclave the mixture at 121 °C for 20 min.
9. 500-mL glass beaker
10. Water bath set to 37 °C.
11. Supplemented medium: DMEM, 40 mM MgCl2, 0.1% cell culture-grade endotoxin-free bovine serum albumin (BSA), 4% FBS.
12. Orbital shaker.
13. Cell culture incubator set at 33 °C, 5% CO2.
14. 4% paraformaldehyde
15. Crystal violet solution: 1% crystal violet, 20% ethanol in water.

2.5 RV-A1B Infection in Immature Mice

1. Vials of RV diluted to 10^8 Plaque-forming units (PFU)/mL with PBS.
2. Six-day-old C57BL/6 or BALB/c mice.
3. Isoflurane/Forane U.S.P.
4. Anesthesia system allowing controlled vaporization of isoflurane.
5. Pipettors and sterilized 20 μl filter tips.
6. Waste container with 10% bleach.

2.6 Lung Tissue Harvesting for Whole Lung RNA Extraction

1. Harvesting tools: small forceps and small scissors.
2. 5-mL sterile syringes with 26 Gauge needle
3. PBS with 0.5 mM EDTA.
4. Round-bottom polypropylene test tubes with cap, 5 mL.
5. TRIzol reagent.
6. Benchtop liquid nitrogen dewar.
7. 70% ethanol

8. Hydrogen peroxide.
9. Handheld tissue homogenizer.

2.7 Processing of Lung Tissue for Flow Cytometry

1. Harvesting tools: small forceps and small scissors.
2. 5 mL sterile syringes with 26 Gauge needle
3. PBS with 0.5 mM EDTA.
4. 100 mm sterile, tissue-culture-treated round culture dishes
5. Flow cytometry digestion buffer: DMEM supplemented with 100 μg/mL Liberase TM, 250 μg/mL collagenase XI, 1 mg/mL hyaluronidase 1a, and 200 μg/mL DNase I.
6. Sterile round-bottom polypropylene test tube with cap, 5 mL.
7. 70-μm nylon mesh cell strainer
8. Sterile 50 mL conical tube.
9. 3 mL syringe
10. Ice-cold PBS with Ca^{2+} and Mg^{2+}.
11. RBC lysis buffer.
12. Resuspension media: DMEM, 100 units/mL of penicillin, 100 μg/mL of streptomycin, 2% FBS.
13. Ice.
14. Rotator.

3 Methods

All procedures for H1HeLa cell culturing and RV-A1B propagation should be performed in a BSL2 biosafety cabinet along with proper personal protective equipment (PPE). All waste from RV-A1B propagation, concentration, and animal infection should be decontaminated with a 10% bleach solution for a minimum of 15 min before disposal.

3.1 H1HeLa Cell Subculturing

1. Seeding H1HeLa cells in a 100 mm cell culture dish. Thaw 1 vial of H1HeLa cells master stock (1 mL; *see* **Note 2**) at 37 ° C. Transfer 1 mL of cell master stock into a sterile 100 mm cell culture dish with 10 mL of H1HeLa media. Place the dish in the incubator set at 37 °C with 5% CO_2 for 16 h.
2. After 16 h, aspirate the spent media off the plate, wash the cells 3 times with 5 mL of PBS (without Ca^{2+} and Mg^{2+}), and add 10 mL of H1HeLa cell media to the dish. Place the dish in the incubator (37 °C, 5% CO_2).
3. Split cells when H1HeLa cells reach confluency of 100%. Wash the cells 3 times with 5 mL of PBS (without Ca^{2+} and Mg^{2+}) by gently rocking the dish to ensure the PBS removes any excess

media and non-viable cells. After aspirating the PBS from the last wash, add 2 mL of 0.25% Trypsin-EDTA solution. Ensure the trypsin-EDTA coats all cells. Place the dish in the incubator (37 °C, 5% CO_2) for 3 min. Tap the side of the dish with your hand to ensure all cells detach.

4. Add 5 mL of H1HeLa media to the dish and mix up the cells by pipetting.
5. Take a small aliquot (50 μL) of H1HeLa cells and mix with trypan blue solution for counting purpose. Count the cells using a hemocytometer.
6. Add 25 mL of fresh H1HeLa media into a new 150 mm cell culture dish and add 1 million cells to the new dish. Place the new dish in the incubator (37 °C, 5% CO_2). Monitor the cells daily till the cells in the 150 mm dish have reached 80–90% confluency.

3.2 RV-A1B Propagation

1. Prepare six 150 mm dishes with 80–90% confluency of H1HeLa cells. Each 150 mm dish will be used to propagate 25 mL of virus-infected stock.
2. Once H1HeLa cells reach 90% of confluency, remove all media from each dish. Add 5 mL of RV-A1B propagation media and 500 ul of RV-A1B master RV-A1B stock (*see* **Note 3**). Place each dish in the incubator (33 °C, 5% CO_2) for 1 h gently rocking the dishes every 15 min.
3. After 1-h incubation, add 20 mL of RV-A1B propagation media into each dish and place all dishes in the incubator (33 °C, 5% CO_2) until 90% of the cells appear to have undergone cytopathic effect (CPE) or have detached from the dish. Monitor cells and CPE daily.
4. When 90% of cells are cytopathic, scrape the plate and collect all viral media-cell mixture. Store the viral media-cell mixture in sterile 50-mL polypropylene conical tubes. Freeze at −70 °C.

3.3 RV-A1B Concentration and Ultrafiltration

1. Thaw the viral media-cell mixture stored in 50-mL conical tubes. Repeat the freeze-thaw twice more.
2. Centrifuge 50-mL conical tubes containing the viral media-cell mixture for 10 min at 10,000× rpm, 4 °C to remove cell debris.
3. In the BSL-2 biosafety cabinet, transfer all viral supernatant (approximately 150 mL from six 150 mm dishes) into a sterile 250 mL vacuum filter unit with a 0.45 μm cellulose acetate membrane. After the filtration, seal and place the collection bottle containing the viral supernatant on ice until ultrafiltration.
4. In the BSL-2 biosafety cabinet, sterilize the Millipore Amicon Stirred Cell (400 mL) ultrafiltration system using 70% ethanol for 15 min. Rinse the ethanol off with sterile PBS three times.

5. Immerse one Millipore Ultracel 100 kDa NMW ultrafiltration disc in 70% ethanol in a 100 mm cell culture dish for 15 min to sterilize. Rinse the ethanol off with sterile PBS three times. Transfer the disc to the bottom plate of the ultrafiltration system with the glossy side up using sterile blunt-end forceps.
6. Assemble the ultrafiltration system in the BSL-2 biosafety cabinet. Add 250 mL of sterile ice-cold PBS with Ca^{2+} and Mg^{2+}. Connect the ultrafiltration system to the pressure regulator tubing of the nitrogen tank in the cold room (4 °C). Facilitate the filtration using a magnetic stirring plate. Apply the pressure to ~40 PSI and wait until the volume drops to 10 mL.
7. Bring the ultrafiltration system to the BSL-2 biosafety cabinet. Add 150 mL of the viral supernatant into the ultrafiltration system. Add RNAse A and DNAse 1 to a final concentration of 10 μg of RNase A per mL and 10 U of DNase1 per mL, and mix well. Connect the ultrafiltration system to the pressure regulator tubing of the nitrogen tank in the cold room (4 °C). Apply the pressure to ~40 PSI and wait until the volume drops to 10 mL.
8. Add 250 mL of sterile ice-cold PBS with Ca^{2+} and Mg^{2+}, and wash the disc by applying pressure.
9. Repeat the PBS washing with 250 mL of sterile ice-cold PBS with Ca^{2+} and Mg^{2+} twice more.
10. Collect the final concentrate (10 mL) and aliquot into cryogenic vials with 1 mL each. Store all the aliquots at −70 °C.
11. Prepare 2 small aliquots with 200 μL of concentrated RV-A1B each for subsequent plaque assay.

3.4 Plaque Assays for Virus Titers

1. Complete Subheading 3.1, **steps 1–5** of the "H1HeLa cell subculturing."
2. Plate H1HeLa cells at 0.5×10^6 cells in 2 mL of H1HeLa media per well in 6-well cell culture plates, 24 h before infection. Each dilution will be assayed in triplicate. Rock the plates left and right, forward and backward, approximately 30 times each to evenly disperse the cells in the well. Do not swirl the plates to avoid the generation of vertex, which pulls the cells to the center of the well.
3. Prepare 1:10 serial dilutions of the viral in virus dilution media. Start the dilutions by adding 1080 μL of cold dilution media to each 1.5 mL microcentrifuge tube. Next, add 120 μL of undiluted virus-infected stock to the first tube (10^{-1} dilution). Vortex this tube well and dispose of the pipette tip into the waste container with 10% bleach. Use a new pipette tip to take 120 μL from the 10^{-1} diluted tube and place it into a second tube with 1080 μL of cold dilution media to make 10^{-2} dilution. Repeat this process to a dilution factor of 10^{-10}. Each well receives 500 μL of the diluted virus.

4. Once all dilutions are ready, take the plates out of the incubator. Aspirate the media from all wells carefully by tilting the plate to one side. Add 500 μL of the diluted virus to each well as planned.
5. Cover the plates and place them on a table rocker for 30 min to allow even adherence of the virus to cells. Next, place the plates in the virus culture-only incubator (33 °C, 5% CO_2) for 30 min.
6. Put the glass ISO bottle (500 mL) containing the prepared 2% SeaPlaque GTG agarose in a glass beaker with water. Microwave or autoclave the agarose to be liquid. Keep the glass bottle-beaker set in the 37 °C water bath. Warm up and keep supplemented medium at 37 °C.
7. In the sterile 50-mL polypropylene conical tubes, mix supplemented medium with 2% agarose at a 1:1 ratio. The final concentration of agarose is 1% agarose.
8. Tilt the plate and aspirate the virus inoculum from the plate edge. Keep tilting the plate and add 4 mL of 1% agarose-supplemented medium mixture to each well at the lower edge of the well.
9. When the agarose has hardened, transfer plates to the humidified incubator (33 °C, 5% CO_2). Monitor CPE and the formation of plaques daily (it takes 3–4 days to see clear plaques).
10. Remove the overlay medium and the agarose layer gently. To accomplish this, overlay the agarose with 2 mL of paraformaldehyde and loosen up the top agarose by nicking the edge of the agarose so that the formalin gets under the agarose layer. Taking a spatula, rim the agarose plug and remove it carefully.
11. Fix the cells with 2 mL of fresh 4% paraformaldehyde solution for 30 min at room temperature.
12. Stain the cells with the freshly prepared crystal violet solution for 10 min at room temperature.
13. After plates are dry, count the plaques of each well and then average the number counted from the three wells in a particular dilution. Plaques typically have relatively uniform edges. Viral titer is determined based on the following formula: the average number of plaques from each dilution × tube dilution factor × 2 = PFU/mL (*see* **Note 4**).

3.5 RV-A1B Infection in Immature Mice

1. Thaw a vial of RV-A1B stock with the titer of 1×10^8 PFU/mL and keep it on ice.
2. Anesthetize a neonatal mouse under the anesthesia system with controlled vaporization of isoflurane via an induction chamber.

3. As soon as an obvious drop in the respiratory rate is observed, the neonatal mouse is ready to be treated intranasally (*see* **Note 5**). Remove the mouse from the chamber and instill 15 μL of RV-A1B (1.5×10^6 PFU) into the mouse intranasally. Continue holding the mouse for a few seconds (*see* **Note 6**).
4. Put the treated neonatal mouse back in the breeding cage. Monitor all mice until they wake up from the anesthesia.

3.6 Lung Tissue Harvesting for Whole Lung RNA Extraction

1. At the designated time point after infection (*see* **Note** 7), add 1 mL of TRIzol reagent into each 5 mL round-bottom polypropylene test tube and keep the tubes on ice.
2. Euthanize the mice using the carbon dioxide exposure method. Once the mouse has been euthanized, place the mouse on the harvesting board with the ventral side up. Pin all four limbs of the mouse to the board, exposing the full ventral side of the mouse and ensuring the skin is taut.
3. Spray the ventral side with 70% ethanol. Use small forceps and small scissors to expose the full thoracic cavity.
4. Perfused lungs with PBS containing 0.5 mM EDTA using a 5-mL sterile syringe with a 26 Gauge needle. Use the forceps to carefully lift the lung and pull it out of the thoracic cavity of the mouse. Use the scissors to cut the connecting tissues attaching the lung to the thoracic cavity.
5. Immediately place the whole lung into the 5 mL tube with 1 mL of TRIzol reagent and snap freeze it by dropping it into a benchtop liquid nitrogen dewar.
6. After removing the lung tissue from the mouse, unpin the mouse and place the carcass into a biohazard bag.
7. Repeat **steps 2–5** for each subsequent bag.
8. Dispose of all biohazard waste and disinfect the harvesting bench. Clean and sanitize all tools with 70% ethanol and hydrogen peroxide.
9. Store all tubes at −70 °C.
10. Thaw the tubes containing the harvested lung tissues and TRIzol. Homogenize the lung tissue using a handheld tissue homogenizer in a BSL-2 biosafety cabinet. Proceed with lung tissue homogenates for subsequent RNA extraction (*see* **Note 8**).

3.7 Processing of Lung Tissue for Flow Cytometry

1. Lung processing for flow cytometry should be performed immediately after harvesting lung tissue from the mouse (*see* **Note 9**).
2. Complete Subheading 3.6, **steps 1–4** of "Lung Tissue Harvesting for Whole Lung RNA Extraction."

3. Use small scissors to finely chop the lungs in a 100 mm cell culture dish. Transfer the chopped lungs to a 5 mL round-bottom polypropylene test tube with 1 mL of digestion buffer. Put the cap on and place all tubes on a rotator. Incubate at room temperature for 1 h.
4. Pour the contents of the 5 mL round-bottom tube over a 70-μm nylon mesh cell strainer on top of a 50 mL conical tube and use the back end of a 3 mL syringe plunger to grind the lung tissue through the cell strainer.
5. Wash the cell strainer and the plunger by pouring 5 mL of sterile PBS with Ca^{2+} and Mg^{2+}. Place the 50 mL conical tube on ice.
6. Repeat **steps 4** and **5** for each sample.
7. Centrifuge all tubes at 1200 rpm for 10 min at 4 °C.
8. Aspirate liquid from each tube.
9. Add 2 mL of 1× RBC lysis buffer to each tube, mix well by pipetting, and place on ice for 5 min.
10. After 5 min, add 8 mL of ice-cold PBS with Ca^{2+} and Mg^{2+} to each tube. Centrifuge all tubes at 1200 rpm for 10 min at 4 °C.
11. Resuspend cells in 2 mL resuspension media. Pour the cells tube over a 70-μm nylon mesh cell strainer on top of a 50 mL conical tube.
12. Take 50 μL of cells for cell counting. Keep the rest of the cells on ice for subsequent flow cytometry staining.

4 Notes

1. 100 kDa NMW ultrafiltration disc is selected because the intact virus particle is too big to go through the 100 kDa cutoff disc.
2. After receiving H1HeLa cells from ATCC, it is required to create H1HeLa master cell stocks with limited passage numbers. The master cell stocks are typically saved in liquid nitrogen tanks. It is also important to keep track of the number of times the cells have been subcultured. Use cells with low passage numbers.
3. After receiving the vial of RV-A1B from ATCC, passage RV-A1B on H1HeLa cells once to generate master RV-A1B virus stocks. The master cell stocks are typically saved in a −70 °C freezer.
4. The viral titer of most RV-A1B-infected stocks prepared in the manner described in Subheadings 3.2 and 3.3 is 5×10^7 PFU/mL to 1×10^9 PFU/mL.
5. Be sure to loosely grab the immature mice and ensure the neck skin is not constricting the airway (Fig. 1). Once the mouse is ready to be treated, remove the mouse from the chamber of the

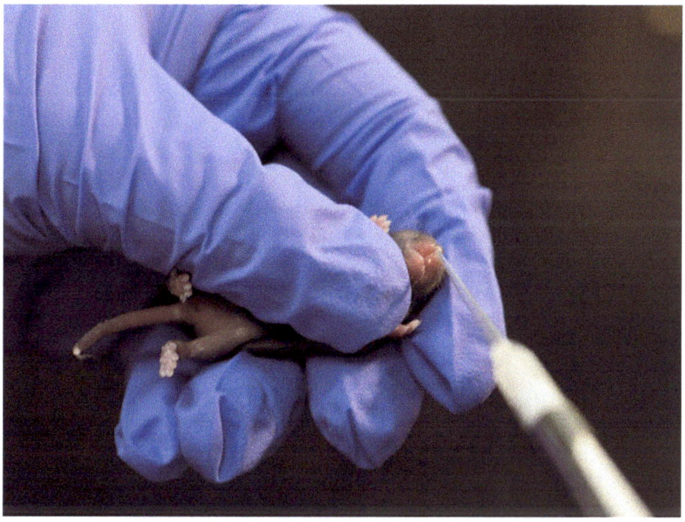

Fig. 1 Intranasal inoculation of RV-A1B into six-day-old immature mice. Anesthetize a six-day-old neonatal mouse under the anesthesia system with controlled vaporization of isoflurane via an induction chamber. As soon as an obvious drop of the respiratory rate is observed, the neonatal mouse is ready to be treated intranasally. Grab the immature mice loosely and gently close the mouth using the thumb. Instill 15 μL of RV-A1B by one or two droplets

anesthesia system and perform the intranasal administration as soon as possible. Overexposure to isoflurane easily leads to the death of immature mice.

6. When infecting mice with RV-A1B, it is common to use a sham infection as a control. The sham infection is carried out using a mock-infected stock that is prepared in the same procedure as the RV-A1B infected stock, just without infection of H1HeLa cells with any RV-A1B. The prepared HeLa cell lysate also goes through 100 kDa NMW ultrafiltration disc.
7. The kinetics for the various outcomes of viral infection are differential. The expression of IL-1β, CXCL-1, CXCL-2, TNF-α, IFN-γ, and IL-33 peaks 1 day after infection, whereas the expression of type 2 cytokines, IL-25, TSLP, and mucin genes, peaks 7 days after infection. PAS staining may peak even later.
8. The whole lung is used for RNA extraction. Lung RNA is extracted following the standard TRIzol protocol and further isolated and purified using a Qiagen RNAeasy kit.
9. Do not snap freeze the lungs if they are to be used in flow cytometry analysis. To determine lung ILCs, lungs are usually harvested 7 or more days post RV-A1B infection in six-day-old mice.

References

1. Hadfield AT, Lee W, Zhao R et al (1997) The refined structure of human rhinovirus 16 at 2.15 a resolution: implications for the viral life cycle. Structure 5:427–441
2. Arruda E, Pitkaranta A, Witek TJ Jr et al (1997) Frequency and natural history of rhinovirus infections in adults during autumn. J Clin Microbiol 35:2864–2868
3. Mosser AG, Brockman-Schneider R, Amineva S et al (2002) Similar frequency of rhinovirus-infectible cells in upper and lower airway epithelium. J Infect Dis 185:734–743
4. Johnston SL, Pattemore PK, Sanderson G et al (1995) Community study of role of viral infections in exacerbations of asthma in 9-11 year old children. BMJ 310:1225–1229
5. Tan WC, Xiang X, Qiu D et al (2003) Epidemiology of respiratory viruses in patients hospitalized with near-fatal asthma, acute exacerbations of asthma, or chronic obstructive pulmonary disease. Am J Med 115:272–277
6. Seemungal T, Harper-Owen R, Bhowmik A et al (2001) Respiratory viruses, symptoms, and inflammatory markers in acute exacerbations and stable chronic obstructive pulmonary disease. Am J Respir Crit Care Med 164:1618–1623
7. Rubner FJ, Jackson DJ, Evans MD et al (2017) Early life rhinovirus wheezing, allergic sensitization, and asthma risk at adolescence. J Allergy Clin Immunol 139:501–507
8. Kotaniemi-Syrjanen A, Vainionpaa R, Reijonen TM et al (2003) Rhinovirus-induced wheezing in infancy – the first sign of childhood asthma? J Allergy Clin Immunol 111:66–71
9. Lemanske RF Jr, Jackson DJ, Gangnon RE et al (2005) Rhinovirus illnesses during infancy predict subsequent childhood wheezing. J Allergy Clin Immunol 116:571–577
10. Jackson DJ, Gangnon RE, Evans MD et al (2008) Wheezing rhinovirus illnesses in early life predict asthma development in high-risk children. Am J Respir Crit Care Med 178: 667–672
11. Jackson DJ, Evans MD, Gangnon RE et al (2012) Evidence for a causal relationship between allergic sensitization and rhinovirus wheezing in early life. Am J Respir Crit Care Med 185:281–285
12. Caliskan M, Bochkov YA, Kreiner-Moller E et al (2013) Rhinovirus wheezing illness and genetic risk of childhood-onset asthma. N Engl J Med 368:1398–1407
13. Bella J, Kolatkar PR, Marlor CW et al (1998) The structure of the two amino-terminal domains of human ICAM-1 suggests how it functions as a rhinovirus receptor and as an LFA-1 integrin ligand. Proc Natl Acad Sci USA 95:4140–4145
14. Vlasak M, Roivainen M, Reithmayer M et al (2005) The minor receptor group of human rhinovirus (HRV) includes HRV23 and HRV25, but the presence of a lysine in the VP1 HI loop is not sufficient for receptor binding. J Virol 79:7389–7395
15. Bartlett NW, Walton RP, Edwards MR et al (2008) Mouse models of rhinovirus-induced disease and exacerbation of allergic airway inflammation. Nat Med 14:199–204
16. Newcomb DC, Sajjan US, Nagarkar DR et al (2008) Human rhinovirus 1B exposure induces phosphatidylinositol 3-kinase-dependent airway inflammation in mice. Am J Respir Crit Care Med 177:1111–1121
17. Schneider D, Hong JY, Popova AP et al (2012) Neonatal rhinovirus infection induces mucous metaplasia and airways hyperresponsiveness. J Immunol 188:2894–2904
18. Hong JY, Bentley JK, Chung Y et al (2014) Neonatal rhinovirus induces mucous metaplasia and airways hyperresponsiveness through IL-25 and type 2 innate lymphoid cells. J Allergy Clin Immunol 134:429–439
19. Han M, Rajput C, Hong JY et al (2017) The innate cytokines IL-25, IL-33, and TSLP cooperate in the induction of type 2 innate lymphoid cell expansion and mucous metaplasia in rhinovirus-infected immature mice. J Immunol 199:1308–1318
20. Han M, Ishikawa T, Bermick JR et al (2020) IL-1beta prevents ILC2 expansion, type 2 cytokine secretion, and mucus metaplasia in response to early-life rhinovirus infection in mice. Allergy 75:2005–2019
21. Han M, Ishikawa T, Stroupe CC et al (2021) Deficient inflammasome activation permits an exaggerated asthma phenotype in rhinovirus C-infected immature mice. Mucosal Immunol 14:1369–1380
22. Han M, Breckenridge HA, Kuo S et al (2022) M2 macrophages promote IL-33 expression, ILC2 expansion and mucous metaplasia in response to early life rhinovirus infections. Front Immunol 13:952509
23. Rajput C, Cui T, Han M et al (2017) RORalpha-dependent type 2 innate lymphoid cells are required and sufficient for mucous metaplasia in immature mice. Am J Physiol Lung Cell Mol Physiol 312:L983–L993
24. Rajput C, Han M, Ishikawa T et al (2020) Early-life heterologous rhinovirus infections induce an exaggerated asthma-like phenotype. J Allergy Clin Immunol 146:571–582

Chapter 15

In Vitro Model to Test Therapeutic Agents Against Rhinovirus Infection

Elizabeth McCluskey and Umadevi Sajjan

Abstract

To develop an antiviral drug, it is extremely important to have a relevant cell culture model system. The airway epithelial cells lining the conductive airways are the primary target for all three classes of rhinoviruses. However, rhinovirus replication is not very robust in airway epithelial cells; therefore, it does not cause cytopathic effects. However, rhinovirus induces replication-dependent cytokines such as type I and type III interferons and CXCL-10, which can be used as surrogates for viral load. Here, we describe a method using the immortalized normal human bronchial epithelial cell line, BEAS-2B cells. These cells readily grow in serum-free medium and can be infected with rhinovirus A and B. The binding, endocytosis, and replication of the virus induce CXCL-8 in these cells. These cells also respond to replicating virus by showing robust CXCL-10 production. Both CXCL-8 and CXCL-10 secreted into the medium can be readily measured by ELISA. Therefore, this method can be used to examine the drugs that can inhibit binding, endocytosis, and replication of the virus.

Key words BEAS-2B cells, CXCL-10, Drug efficacy

1 Introduction

Respiratory tract infections (RTIs) are the most common type of acute infection globally in both adults and children [1]. Rhinoviruses (RV) cause self-limiting upper respiratory infections globally and are the major cause of common colds in healthy individuals [2]. The economic impact of RV infection is huge because of both sick days and purchasing of non-prescription drugs to relieve the cold symptoms. In 2003, the annual expenses related to common cold were estimated at $40 billion in the US alone, and this may be much higher globally. In patients with chronic respiratory illnesses such as asthma, cystic fibrosis (CF), and chronic obstructive pulmonary disease (COPD), rhinovirus infection is associated with acute exacerbations, which can often lead to the progression of lung disease [1, 3]. This further increases the economic burden globally. So far, there are no effective vaccines or drugs for the

Umadevi Sajjan (ed.), *Rhinovirus: Methods and Protocols*, Methods in Molecular Biology, vol. 2903,
https://doi.org/10.1007/978-1-0716-4410-2_15,

treatment of rhinovirus infection. Therefore, the search for new antiviral drugs and therapeutic agents against rhinovirus is crucial. Almost all viruses encode unique proteins and enzymes that designed compounds may specifically target in order to inhibit viral entry or viral replication [4].

There are more than 160 serotypes of RV identified to date, and phylogenetically, they are categorized into three groups: RV-A, RV-B, and RV-C [5–7]. The majority of viruses in the RV-A and RV-B groups enter the cells by binding to human ICAM-1, while others bind to low-density lipoprotein (LDL) receptors or LDL receptor-like proteins [8, 9] and cadherin-related family member 3 (CDHR3) [10]. RV-A and RV-B effectively infect and replicate in H1HeLa cells, and therefore these cells have been used to screen the potential drug candidates in this cell line. RV-C infects and replicates only in mucociliary differentiated human airway epithelium. In previous studies, a full-length RV-C replicon chimera expressing luciferase was transfected into H1HeLA cells to determine the antiviral efficacy of selected drugs [11].

Replication of RV-A and RV-B viruses causes cytopathic effects in H1HeLa cells [12]. Therefore, for screening antiviral drugs, investigators quantify the cytopathic effect when using H1HeLa cells. Although several potential antiviral drugs have been identified using this cell line, none of these molecules are currently used in the clinic to treat RV infections. This suggests that these drugs may not be effective in blocking viral entry or replication in airway epithelial cells, which are the primary targets for RV. Therefore, it is necessary to use airway epithelial cells as an in vitro model system for screening anti-rhinoviral drugs.

RV infection does not cause cytopathic effects in airway epithelial cells; therefore, we propose an assay other than cytotoxicity should be used to screen the efficacy of the antiviral drug. Mucociliary-differentiated airway epithelial cell culture is the best in vitro model for investigating on innate immune responses to RV infection, but it may not be suitable for screening drugs because of the variable responses of cells from one donor to another, as well as the cost and the time required for culturing the cells. The epithelial cell lines 16HBE14o- cells and BEAS-2B cells were derived from normal bronchial cells. The 16HBE14o- cells polarize and are useful for determining the RV-induced disruption of barrier function, but unlike primary cells, they do not show robust innate immune responses to RV. On the other hand, BEAS-2B cells do not polarize but show robust innate immune responses to RV infection and could be useful in screening the drugs. The assay of choice to test the efficacy in these cells should be either the quantification of viral load or replicating virus-induced responses such as CXCL-10, type I, and type III interferons. Quantification of viral load is rather labor-intensive unless the recombinant rhinovirus expressing a fluorophore is used. Recently, an RV-1A construct expressing green fluorescent protein or iLOV was generated, and the latter was demonstrated to infect H1HeLa cells [13]. However, infection of cells with the recombinant virus was lower than the parent strain, and in airway epithelial cells, the fluorescent signals could not be detected, questioning the utility of this recombinant virus in drug screening. Conversely, CXCL-8, stimulated by the binding/endocytosis/replication of the virus, or CXCL-10, stimulated by replicating virus, could be readily measured in the cell culture medium by ELISA and can be automated. In this chapter, we provide a method for screening the antiviral drugs using the BEAS-2B epithelial cell line.

2 Materials

1. BEAS-2B cell line (ATCC CRL-9609, Manassas, VA).
2. Bronchial cell growth medium bullet kit (BEGM) (CC-3170, Lonza, Walkerville, MD). The medium can also be prepared in the lab following the protocol previously described [14]. For the preparation of medium components, see Chapter 9 (*see* **Note 1**).
   (a) 500 mL LHC basal medium (ThermoFisher Scientific Cat# 12677019)
   (b) 5 mL L-glutamine (ThermoFisher Scientific Cat# A2916801)
   (c) 5 mL Penicillin/Streptomycin (ThermoFisher Scientific Cat# 15140122)
   (d) 1× trace elements (see Chapter 9)
   (e) 1× stock 4 salt solution (see Chapter 9)
   (f) Cell culture grade BSA 0.5 mg/mL (see Chapter 9).
   (g) 2 mL bovine pituitary extract with total protein content of 13 mg/mL (see Chapter 9)
   (h) Insulin 0.125 μM
   (i) Transferrin 0.125 μM
   (j) Epidermal growth factor 12.5 ng/mL
   (k) Hydrocortisone 0.1 μg/mL
   (l) Triiodothyronine 0.01 μM
   (m) Epinephrine 2.7 μM
   (n) Retinoic acid s $\times 10^{-8}$ M
   (o) Phosphorylethanolmine 0.5 μM
   (p) Ethanolamine 0.5 μM
3. Bovine type I collagen (Advanced BioMatrix, Carlsbad, CA).

4. 100 mm × 15 mm tissue-culture treated plates.
5. Flat bottom tissue-culture treated 96-well plates.
6. Rhinovirus stocks RV16 (ATCC VR-283), RV1B (ATCC VR-1648)—propagated in H1HeLa cell followed by ultrafiltration (please refer to Chapter 2 in this book).
7. Infection medium (BEGM with no hydrocortisone).
8. Cell storage medium (BEGM, 10% DMSO, 10% fetal bovine serum).
9. Sterile cell culture grade PBS without $CaCl_2$ and $MgCl_2$.
10. Trypsin/EDTA: 0.25% (w/v) trypsin/0.02% (w/v) EDTA (Gibco 25200056 or equivalent).
11. Humidified, 37 °C, 5% CO_2 incubator.
12. Humidified, 33 °C, 5% CO_2 incubator.
13. Water bath set to 37 °C.
14. −80 °C freezer.
15. Liquid nitrogen tank.
16. Biosafety Level 2 cell culture hood.
17. A benchtop refrigerated centrifuge.
18. Sterile 15-mL conical centrifuge tubes.
19. Sterile 50-mL conical centrifuge tubes.
20. Sterile 5, 10, 25 mL serological pipettes.
21. Sterile 2-mL cryovials.
22. Hemacytometer.
23. Ethanol 70%.
24. Multichannel pipette (250 μL).
25. Sterile polystyrene reagent reservoir (Corning/Costar #CLS4870 or equivalent).
26. CXCL-8 and CXCL-10 duoset ELISA kits (Bio-Techne Cat# DY208 and DY266).
27. Spectrophotometer to read 96 wells.

3 Methods

3.1 Coating of Cell Culture Dishes with Collagen

Coat 10 cm tissue culture plates with collagen at 5 μg/cm^2. Dilute collagen in sterile distilled water and add 7 mL containing 293 μg of collagen to 10 cm dishes. For 96-well plates, add 0.5 μg of collagen diluted in 50 μL of sterile distilled water. Incubate overnight at 4 °C or 4–6 h at room temperature water. Aspirate and UV-irradiate the plates in the cell culture hood for 45 min to 1 h.

Before plating the cells, wash the plates twice with sterile distilled water and remove all traces of water.

3.2 Expansion of BEAS-2B Cells

1. Warm up sufficient BEGM in a 37 °C water bath for 20 min. Typically, 10 mL medium/one 10 cm dish. Rinse the outside of the tube and transfer it to the hood.
2. Wash collagen-coated plate with sterile distilled water and remove all traces of water and add 10 mL warm medium.
3. Thaw a vial of BEAS-2B cells (approximately 1×10^6 cells) in a water bath for 1–2 min. Rinse the outside of the vial with 70% alcohol. Transfer to the cell culture hood and immediately add to a 10 cm dish containing warm medium dropwise. Rinse the tube with 1 mL of warm medium and add it to the 10-cm dish. Incubate in a cell culture incubator until the cells reach 80% confluency. Change the medium on alternate days.
4. Trypsinization and storage of cells: Once the cells are 80% confluent, aspirate medium and wash cells with warm PBS twice. Add 2 mL trypsin/EDTA, incubate at 37 °C for 2 min and then 3–5 min at RT. Collect the cells into a 50 mL tube containing 0.5 mL FBS. Rinse the plate with PBS to collect all the cells. Centrifuge at 500× *g* for 5 min. Aspirate supernatant and suspend the pellet in 4 mL BEGM, count the cells, and add serum and DMSO to 10% each. Aliquot cell suspension at a density of 1–2 × 10^6 cells/ml in cryovials and store in liquid nitrogen tank.
5. Use the cells at early passage number (between 2 and 8) to obtain reproducible results (*see* **Note 2**).
6. BEAS-2B cells may contain mycoplasma and therefore cells must be tested for mycoplasma routinely (*see* **Note 3**).

3.3 Rhinovirus Infection of Cells

1. Seeding cells in 96-well plate: Grow the cells in a 10 cm dish as mentioned above, trypsinize the cells, and suspend the cell pellet in BEGM so that the density of the cell suspension is 1×10^5 cell/mL. Transfer the cell suspension to a sterile polystyrene disposable reservoir and add 100 uL to each well with a multichannel pipette.
2. Incubate for 24 h at 37 °C.
3. Aspirate the medium and infect cells with 30 μL of medium containing rhinovirus (1×10^5 pfu; the multiplicity of infection at 5).
4. Incubate for 2 h at 37 °C to promote the virus to bind and enter the cells.
5. Add 70 uL of medium and continue incubation for another 22 h at 33 °C.
6. Centrifuge the plate at 1000× *g* for 10 min at 4 °C.

7. The supernatant is analyzed for CXCL-8 and CXCL-10 immediately or can be stored at −80 °C for up to 2 weeks.

3.4 Treatment with Antiviral Drugs

1. If the antiviral drugs are targeted to inhibit binding or endocytosis of rhinovirus, incubate the cells with varying concentrations of drug prior to the addition of rhinovirus overnight or for 2 h. The culture medium containing drugs should be used for infection and replenishing the medium after infection.
2. If the antiviral drugs are targeted to inhibit replication of the virus after the virus is endocytosed, add the cell culture medium containing various concentrations of the antiviral drug after infection.
3. Incubated the cells for 8–24 h.
4. Collect the medium, centrifuge, and collect the supernatant.
5. Uninfected cells treated with drug or placebo must be used as controls (*see* **Note 4**).

3.5 CXCL-10 and CXCL-8 ELISA

1. If the supernatants are frozen, thaw them on ice.
2. Mix gently by pipetting or vortexing at low speed.
3. Determine the levels of CXCL-10 and CXCL-8 by ELISA following the manufacturer's instructions (*see* **Note 5**).

The cells that are not infected with rhinovirus show no detectable CXCL-10 protein and very little CXCL-8 in the cell culture supernatant. In response to dsRNA generated during rhinovirus replication stimulates expression of abundant CXCL-10 ranging from 100 to 1000 pg/mL, which can be readily detected by ELISA. The cells produce CXCL-8 in response to viral binding, endocytosis, and replication, and it ranges from 2 to 4 ng/mL. The drugs with antiviral effects or which inhibits binding and endocytosis will reduce the expression of CXCL-10 and CXCL-8 significantly.

4 Notes

1. If using a large amount of medium, home-made medium is cheaper and gives more reproducible results than the commercially available medium.
2. Please note that at higher passage numbers, the cells change the morphology and look more like fibroblasts. These cells show abnormal responses to rhinovirus infection.
3. The presence of mycoplasma may increase the levels of CXCL-8 and induce CXCL-10 under unstimulated conditions. In addition, mycoplasma-containing cells do not show optimal response to rhinovirus. Therefore, it is important to test the

cells for mycoplasma contamination prior to using the cells. The cells should be also tested for mycoplasma routinely.

4. The drug or placebo by themselves may affect the integrity of the cells, which can stimulate CXCL-8 or kill the cells. Therefore, it is important to include the uninfected controls treated with drug and placebo at a concentration that will be used to test the antiviral capacity of the drug in infected cells.
5. It may be necessary to dilute the culture medium, particularly for the determination of CXCL-8 from RV-infected cell cultures, by ten-fold.

References

1. Gaunt E, Harvala H, McIntyre C, Templeton K, Simmonds P (2011) Disease burden of the most commonly detected respiratory viruses in hospitalized patients calculated using the disability adjusted life year (DALY) model. J Clin Virol 52:215–221
2. Makela MJ, Puhakka T, Ruuskanen O, Leinonen M, Saikku P, Kimpimaki M, Blomqvist S, Hyypia T, Arstila P (1998) Viruses and bacteria in the etiology of the common cold. J Clin Microbiol 36:539–542
3. Rijsbergen LC, Van Dijk LL, Engel MF, De Vries RD, De Swart RL (2021) In vitro modelling of respiratory virus infections in human airway epithelial cells–a systematic review. Front Immunol 3301
4. Rumlová M, Ruml T (2018) In vitro methods for testing antiviral drugs. Biotechnol Adv 36: 557–576
5. Palmenberg AC, Spiro D, Kuzmickas R, Wang S, Djikeng A, Rathe JA, Fraser-Liggett CM, Liggett SB (2009) Sequencing and analyses of all known human rhinovirus genomes reveal structure and evolution. Science 324: 55–59
6. McErlean P, Shackelton LA, Andrews E, Webster DR, Lambert SB, Nissen MD, Sloots TP, Mackay IM (2008) Distinguishing molecular features and clinical characteristics of a putative new rhinovirus species, human rhinovirus C (HRV C). PLoS One 3:e1847
7. McIntyre CL, McWilliam Leitch EC, Savolainen-Kopra C, Hovi T, Simmonds P (2010) Analysis of genetic diversity and sites of recombination in human rhinovirus species C. J Virol 84:10297–10310
8. Smith TJ, Kremer MJ, Luo M, Vriend G, Arnold E, Kamer G, Rossmann MG, McKinlay MA, Diana GD, Otto MJ (1986) The site of attachment in human rhinovirus 14 for antiviral agents that inhibit uncoating. Science 233:1286–1293
9. Uncapher CR, DeWitt CM, Colonno RJ (1991) The major and minor group receptor families contain all but one human rhinovirus serotype. Virology 180:814–817
10. Bochkov YA, Watters K, Ashraf S, Griggs TF, Devries MK, Jackson DJ, Palmenberg AC, Gern JE (2015) Cadherin-related family member 3, a childhood asthma susceptibility gene product, mediates rhinovirus C binding and replication. Proc Natl Acad Sci USA 112: 5485–5490
11. Mello C, Aguayo E, Rodriguez M, Lee G, Jordan R, Cihlar T, Birkus G (2014) Multiple classes of antiviral agents exhibit in vitro activity against human rhinovirus type C. Antimicrob Agents Chemother 58:1546–1555
12. Kaiser L, Crump CE, Hayden FG (2000) In vitro activity of pleconaril and AG7088 against selected serotypes and clinical isolates of human rhinoviruses. Antivir Res 47:215–220
13. Han M, Rajput C, Hinde JL, Wu Q, Lei J, Ishikawa T, Bentley JK, Hershenson MB (2018) Construction of a recombinant rhinovirus accommodating fluorescent marker expression. Influenza Other Respir Viruses 12:717–727
14. Fulcher ML, Gabriel S, Burns KA, Yankaskas JR, Randell SH (2005) Well-differentiated human airway epithelial cell cultures. Methods Mol Med 107:183–206

Index

A

Adherens junctions (AJs) 77
Adoptive transfer 154, 161
Airway basal cells 97, 98, 101, 103, 107
Airway epithelial cells (AECs) 9, 17, 29, 31, 32, 40, 52, 65–75, 77–95, 106, 143, 153, 186, 187
Airway epithelium 22, 97, 98, 105, 110, 149, 153, 186
Apical junctional complexes (AJCs) 77–79, 81–85, 87–94
Asthma 9, 21, 22, 31, 65, 86, 90, 91, 98, 114, 141–143, 151, 153–161, 173–183, 185

B

Barrier disruption 78, 114
BEAS-2B cells 186, 189
Bronchoalveolar lavage (BAL) 2, 167, 169

C

Carboxyfluorescein diacetate succinimydyl methyl ester (CFSE) 155, 161
Cell death 32, 109, 121–123
Chronic obstructive pulmonary disease (COPD) 9, 21, 31, 65, 97–107, 109, 110, 141, 143, 151, 165–170, 173, 185
Confocal microscopy 81, 89, 95, 133–137
Crystal violet 32, 34, 36–38, 66, 67, 72, 74, 176, 180
CXCL-10 147, 151, 186–188, 190
Cytokines 17, 28, 29, 98, 107, 114, 125–133, 147, 151, 153, 169, 174, 183

D

Detection 2–4, 7, 17, 27, 31, 50, 63, 85, 119, 125, 126, 130–132, 142
Drug efficacy 142

E

Early-life 153, 173, 174
Elastase 166–170
Emphysema 166, 169, 170
Endosomes 52, 55, 60, 62, 63
Epithelial barrier 78, 114, 123
Epithelial permeability 78, 79, 87, 121

F

Flow cytometry 51–63, 154, 156–159, 169, 177, 181–183

G

Group 2 innate lymphoid cells (ILC2s) 153, 154, 157–161, 174

H

H1HeLa cells 10–14, 17, 18, 22, 32, 34, 37, 38, 52, 65, 73, 143, 166, 167, 174, 175, 177–179, 182, 183, 186, 187
HeLa cells 10, 22–24, 26, 27, 32, 34, 51, 52, 156, 183
Human rhinovirus 1, 21, 65

I

Immunofluorescence (IF) 80–81, 116, 133–137, 149–151, 154, 160–161
In-Cell Western™ 79–80, 83
Inflammation 10, 110, 142, 148, 150, 166, 169, 174
Innate immunity 97, 98, 110, 113, 186
Interferons 28, 107, 147, 151, 186

L

Lineage negative cells 159
Lymphocytes 153, 158

M

Methods 1–6, 10, 12–17, 22–29, 34–37, 39–49, 52–62, 66–73, 78, 81–93, 98, 103–107, 116–137, 143–151, 154, 156–161, 167–169, 174, 177–182, 187–190
Microtiter plate 66, 72, 75

Umadevi Sajjan (ed.), *Rhinovirus: Methods and Protocols*, Methods in Molecular Biology, vol. 2903,
https://doi.org/10.1007/978-1-0716-4410-2,

Mouse 10, 17, 29, 32, 52, 53, 80, 110, 129, 130, 135, 142–144, 147–161, 165–170, 173–183
Mucociliary differentiation 27, 106
Mucus secretion 148, 151, 166

N

Nasal epithelium.................................113, 142, 149–151
Negative-strand RNAs 39–50

R

Real-time PCR 1, 2, 4, 6, 40, 42–50, 142, 147
Real-time PCR genomic RNA 39–50
Receptors 9, 10, 22, 32, 40, 42, 51, 52, 78, 79, 113, 121, 124–125, 143, 153, 157, 158, 173, 186
Rhinovirus (RV)........................1, 11, 21, 31, 39, 51, 65, 78, 98, 113, 141, 153, 165, 173, 185
Rhinovirus antibody.. 52

S

Super-resolution microscopy...................................88, 91

T

Tight junctions (TJs) 77, 86, 90, 91
Tissue culture infectivity dose 50 ($TCID_{50}$) 32, 41, 43, 49, 66, 71–73, 75
Transepithelial electrical resistance (TEER) 78, 85, 86
Transfection 23, 26, 27
Type 2 immune response..174

U

Ultracentrifugation 22, 99
Ultrafiltration 10, 11, 15, 17–19, 22, 23, 26, 28, 143, 150, 175, 178–179, 182, 183, 188

V

Viral infections 51, 78, 110, 114, 119–121, 123, 153, 166, 174, 183
Viral purification 9–19, 168
Viral titers 14, 36, 37, 39, 40, 65, 67, 72, 73, 119, 176, 180, 182
Virus infectivity assay

W

Wheeze 114
WI-38 fibroblasts 67, 68

MIX
Papier aus verantwortungsvollen Quellen
Paper from responsible sources
FSC® C105338

If you have any concerns about our products,
you can contact us on
ProductSafety@springernature.com

In case Publisher is established outside the EU,
the EU authorized representative is:
Springer Nature Customer Service Center GmbH
Europaplatz 3, 69115 Heidelberg, Germany

Printed by Libri Plureos GmbH
in Hamburg, Germany